Blood Pressure

Self-Measurement

Dr. J. Morley

Morden Books

First published in Great Britain 2009
by Morden Books

Disclaimer

This book provides information for educational purposes only. It is not intended as, and does not substitute for, medical advice. It will enable individuals and patients to understand the measurement of high blood pressure. If you are a patient, please see your doctor for evaluation of your individual case. It is essential to consult a medical adviser in order to diagnose and treat high blood pressure. The author and publishers therefore disclaim all liability for direct or consequential damages resulting from the use of material contained in this publication. Readers are strongly advised to pay careful attention to information provided by the manufacturer of any drug or equipment that they plan to use.

ISBN: 978-0-9563318-0-9

For additional information visit www.self-measurement.co.uk

Printed in Great Britain by the MPG Books Group, Bodmin and King's Lynn

Contents

1. Summary

High blood pressure is also known as hypertension. It is a chronic illness that lacks symptoms and can only be diagnosed by regular measurement of arterial pressure. In developed countries, nine out of ten individuals will experience high blood pressure at some point during their lives and, by damaging brain, heart or kidney, this condition will ultimately cause death in half of the population. Before treatment became available, it was presumed that high blood pressure improved the perfusion of organs that had been damaged by vascular disease. Hence, high blood pressure was for many years described as "essential hypertension". However, when drugs were used to lower blood pressure, this perception was confounded by a reduced incidence of both strokes and heart attacks.

When arterial vessels of the heart, brain, and kidneys are damaged by high pressure, the only simple indication is a raised blood pressure. Overestimation (white coat hypertension) or underestimation (masked hypertension) can obscure this effect if pressures are measured in a medical setting. Self-measurement eliminates these errors and thereby provides a more sensitive method for detecting the organ damage that precedes a stroke or a coronary heart attack. Such damage commences once usual blood pressures exceed 115 (systolic) or 75 (diastolic) mm of mercury. Hence, it is worthwhile to use self-measurement before diagnosis of high blood pressure at 140 (systolic) or 90 (diastolic) mm of mercury. After diagnosis regular self-measurement ensures close control of blood pressure and is of especial value to patients who are diabetic or who have previously experienced a stroke or a coronary heart attack.

Anyone making regular measurements of blood pressure will become aware of considerable variation between replicate measurements. Since the body experiences surges of pressure whenever there is any physical activity, changes of pressure variation are inevitable. Understandably therefore, usual blood pressure cannot be revealed by an isolated measurement. To define usual blood pressure with any certainty, successive measurements have to be averaged over several days. This may seem laborious; but it is more practicable and convenient than attempting successive visits to a clinic. Self-measurement is therefore the preferred method for securing the regular measurements needed for satisfactory control of blood pressure.

Persisting high blood pressure underlies the strokes and coronary heart attacks that are commonplace in developed countries. There is a high prevalence of both conditions amongst the elderly. Hence, it is widely presumed that strokes and coronary heart attacks must be inescapable consequences of ageing. However, there are isolated communities in which blood pressure is not raised and does not increase with age. In these communities, strokes or coronary heart attacks occur rarely, if ever; yet, on adopting an urban lifestyle their vulnerability rises progressively until it matches our own. From this, it can be inferred that it is not because of the aging process that strokes and coronary heart attacks are prevalent amongst the elderly. Rather, it is because the damage produced by protracted exposure to high blood pressure is cumulative and irreversible.

The clear association between lifestyle in isolated communities and an absence of high blood pressure raises the possibility that adopting such a lifestyle in developed countries could retard, or even avert, onset of high blood pressure. Certainly, it is reasonable to expect that exercising regularly and eating sparingly could prevent an upward drift of blood pressure in young adults. The same outcome is less likely in middle-age. In all probability, the middle aged will have progressed already into pre-hypertension. Furthermore, it is likely that their eating habits will have become ingrained and their capacity for vigorous exercise will be limited by restricted mobility. It is therefore unlikely that diet and exercise can be used to retard upward progression of blood pressure in the middle-aged, unless augmented by pharmaceuticals.

The World Health Organisation anticipates that vascular disease will become the leading cause of death in developed countries by 2020. This epidemic almost certainly reflects a lifestyle in which there is excessive consumption of animal fats, refined carbohydrates and salt, use of machines for transportation and avoidance of muscular efforts that are intense or protracted, as well as close control of the environment within dwellings, offices and factories. Within these communities, the prevalence of high blood pressure predisposes to coronary heart attacks and strokes. Because coronary heart attacks are the commonest cause of premature death in adults and because two thirds of stroke victims will either die or experience persisting disability, it is imperative to avert progression towards high blood pressure. Now that electronic recorders of blood pressure have prices that are comparable with bathroom scales, it is likely that self-measurement of blood pressure will become as routine as measurement of body weight. Monitoring these aspects of body function by self-measurement is simple and should enable you to avoid much of the ill health that stems from damage to arterial vessels.

If you decide to measure your own blood pressure, you should follow protocols that ensure reliable measurement. To obtain averages of sufficient precision, paired measurements must be recorded each morning and evening for a minimum of seven successive days. Such averages can detect high blood pressure and will establish whether control of blood pressure is adequate. Before the onset of high blood pressure, routine self-measurement will detect any upward trend and alert you to the possibility of covert damage to vital organs. For discussion with your doctor, it is essential to have clear and concise summaries of your measurements. Hence, in addition to explaining the methodology of blood pressure measurement as well as the origin, consequences and treatment of high blood pressure, this book suggests ways to record your measurements that can be appraised rapidly by your doctor.

2. High blood pressure

2.1   Why does blood circulate under pressure?

- Circulating blood supplies oxygen and nutrients to tissues and concurrently removes carbon dioxide and other toxic wastes
- Exchange of these materials occurs as blood passes through very fine tubes that permeate tissues
- High pressures are needed to overcome a high resistance to flow in these fine tubes
- High pressure is produced by contraction of the heart and is sustained between contractions by elasticity of the arterial wall
- As well as ensuring rapid exchange of materials within tissues, high arterial pressure facilitates high flow rates in lungs, liver and kidneys

It is not self-evident why our blood should circulate under high pressure. After all, most organisms are able to prosper despite an absence of blood. Plants do not contain blood; nor do the majority of invertebrate animals. In all plants and in the majority of animal species, those chemicals upon which life depends enter or leave the body simply by diffusing along gradients of chemical concentration. In most organisms, this process of diffusion supplies oxygen and nutrients in adequate amounts and eliminates carbon dioxide and other waste materials. Animals that maintain very closely controlled conditions within the body utilise blood for transportation of gases around the body in order to evade limitations imposed by simple diffusion.

Exchange of gases and other chemicals is achieved by diffusion across the outer surface of simple organisms. Over distances of < 1 mm, diffusion provides sufficient oxygen for metabolic needs. The constraint of diffusion therefore limits the size, and controls the shape, of simple organisms. One way of circumventing this restriction is to transport gases into the tissues. For instance, oxygen will diffuse more deeply into tissues if it is transported as a gas along fine air-filled tubes. This method of delivery is used by insects to extend the range of diffusion of gases, effectively by several mm. Even so, the largest insects are smaller than the vast majority of vertebrate species.

Some invertebrates and all vertebrates escape the constraints of diffusion by using a special fluid to transport gases around the body. In aquatic organisms, concentrations of gases within vessels that lie close to the body surface are closely similar to concentrations within the surrounding water. The fluid used to transport gases through these vessels is frequently adapted to transport large amounts of oxygen. By this means, tissue deep within the body can be exposed to concentrations of oxygen that match those at the body surface. The counterpart of diffusion of oxygen into tissues is a diffusion of carbon dioxide away from tissues. Hence, there is concurrent elimination of carbon dioxide from the body surface. Although the common frog has lungs, these animals often rely on diffusion across the skin to achieve gas exchange, as when at rest. The maximum rate of exchange of gases across skin is insufficient for the metabolic needs of animals that are larger or more active. To overcome this limitation, specialised structures (i.e. gills, lungs) are used to exchange gases between blood and the external environment. Within these structures, diffusion over distances approaching 1mm would achieve equilibrium far too slowly. Hence, blood is transported through these structures within a mesh of very fine, thin-walled tubing within which rates of diffusion of gases are not limiting. A similar network of capillaries is used to exchange of gases within tissues throughout the body. Multi-chambered pumps (i.e. hearts) provide the high pressures that are needed to ensure high rates of flow through these two populations of very fine vessels. Such high-pressure systems have evolved independently in crustaceans (e.g. crab, lobster), molluscs (e.g. squid, cuttlefish) and vertebrates (e.g. fish, amphibians, reptiles, birds, mammals).

When body temperature matches environmental temperatures, relatively low perfusion pressures may provide amounts of oxygen that are adequate for movement and intermittent feeding will suffice for most metabolic needs. The rate of tissue growth will be a limitation and reduces the rate and frequency of reproduction. Birds and mammals avoid this constraint by maintaining a constant, relatively high, internal body temperature. As well as allowing the rapid growth needed for reproduction, a high body temperature enables animals to move rapidly for long periods regardless of the environmental temperature. Birds and mammals therefore require a high rate of blood flow not only for gas exchange and for elimination of wastes but also for mobilisation of stored energy when adequate food supplies are unavailable. To achieve this objective, heat and nutrient materials are transferred from skeletal muscle and liver before being propelled into the lungs for enrichment with oxygen and to the kidneys and liver for elimination of toxic materials. This ensures that tissues throughout the body receive a constant supply of oxygen and nutrients in warm, preconditioned blood. In warm-blooded animals, use of high-pressure tissue perfusion will guarantee a continuous supply of large quantities of such preconditioned blood to the brain and heart. The need for continuous supply of preconditioned blood can be made obvious by causing an abrupt cessation of blood flow. For instance, interruption of flow to the human brain produces a loss of consciousness within five seconds and progresses to irreversible damage within minutes.

In human adults, one litre of blood must flow through the brain and heart every minute to provide an adequate supply of oxygen. These flow rates are very high and almost match flow rates to the liver and kidneys. For this reason, as much as 70% of the output from the heart enters brain, heart, liver and kidneys, even though they comprise less than 5% of total body weight (See Table 1).

Organ	Weight (kg)	Blood flow (litres/min)	Perfusion (litres/kg/min)
Brain	1.5	0.75	0.5
Heart	0.3	0.15	0.5
Liver	1.5	1.5	1.0
Kidneys	0.3	1.2	4.0
Muscles	25.0	0.75	0.03
Other organs & tissues	40.0	0.65	0.015
Whole body	68.6	5.0	0.075

Table 1. Distribution of blood flow in the organs and tissues of an adult at rest

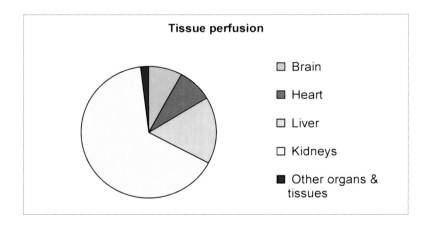

Figure 1. Perfusion of organs and tissues by blood in an adult at rest

Figure 1 illustrates how blood is distributed on leaving the heart. Most will be routed to the liver and kidney, with a lesser amount being delivered to the heart and brain. When the body is at rest, flow of blood through skeletal muscles, bone, gut, glands and other tissues remains inconsequential since these tissues require only modest amounts of oxygen whilst inactive. In the case of skeletal muscle, it is only during contraction and recovery that oxygen is used in increasing amounts and carbon dioxide released in quantity. During contraction, the flow of blood through skeletal muscle rises abruptly and can increase by up to 20-fold within a minute. Corresponding changes of flow occur when digestive glands are producing secretions. For instance, copious amounts of fluid have to be transferred from blood into collecting ducts to allow tenacious secretions to be expelled from salivary glands. For this reason, flow of blood in the salivary gland may increase by up to 100-fold within seconds, which enables cat to spit during fighting. This massive bulk transfer of water matches that in the collecting tubules of the kidney during formation of urine. Not surprisingly therefore, maximal rates of blood flow in a salivary gland during secretion match the high rates of blood flow that are characteristic of mammalian kidney.

It is imperative that supplies of oxygen and nutrients to the brain and heart are not diminished whenever there are changes of blood flow within other parts of the body. The brain and the heart use large amounts of oxygen continuously and are sensitive to accumulated metabolic wastes as well as to any reduction of nutrients. Consequently, even a slight reduction of blood flow can produce serious malfunction in either organ. For this reason, pressure within major arterial vessels is held above a minimum value. Such close control of blood pressure is achieved by using sensors to monitor blood pressure continuously within the large vessels that supply these organs. On detecting any slight fall of pressure, processes are initiated that restore lost pressure and pre-empt any further fall of pressure. Because loss of perfusion pressure can rapidly be fatal, overlapping control systems are used to maintain blood pressure and to guarantee constant perfusion of vital organs.

When the output of blood from the heart is increased or when there is a selective increase of resistance to flow in small arteries throughout the body, arterial blood pressure will rise. For instance, the rate of delivery of blood from the heart will increased if its chambers are allowed to fill to a greater extent before expulsion of blood and/or if there is increased frequency of contraction. By these means, the amount of blood delivered to active tissues can increase by up to seven-fold without compromising flow to the brain or heart muscle. Alternatively, blood pressure may be maintained by causing arterial vessels to narrow, which increases their resistance to the flow of blood. In tissues that are poorly tolerant of a reduced blood supply, vessel narrowing is selectively curtailed. For tissues such that can tolerate very low rates of perfusion, as in the skin, reduced flow can be very protracted.

The overriding objective of mechanisms that compensate for reduced blood pressure is to maintain flow of blood into the brain and heart, effectively on pain of death. These mechanisms have evolved to increase our chances of survival during severe injury. Such emergencies are now relatively infrequent. Hence, increased blood pressure has become a mixed blessing since the advantage of minimising acute injury has to be set against damage caused by protracted high blood pressure. Persisting high blood pressure is disadvantageous because of the increased risk of activating the clotting cascade and causing platelets to clump within small arteries. As high blood pressure occurs predominantly in later life, traits that favour this condition are not readily eliminated from the population.

2.2   How is blood pressure measured?

- For direct measurement, a fluid filled tube is introduced into an artery and connected to a pressure transducer
- For indirect measurement, blood flow in an extremity is prevented by an inflated cuff whose pressure changes are monitored as blood flow is restored
- For clinical studies, indirect measurements are preferred since replication causes minimal discomfort and no damage

Blood that is to be distributed into tissues is held under pressure inside arterial vessels that are encased within a tough fibrous sheath. Because this sheath is relatively inflexible, the dimensions of arteries do not change appreciably as arterial pressure rises. Consequently, the physical appearance of those arteries that are visible just beneath the skin does not change when blood pressure rises. It is this lack of any physical indication of high blood pressure that makes regular measurement mandatory for diagnosis and treatment of high blood pressure.

Arterial pressure can be measured directly by using a fluid-filled tube to attach a manometer to the cut end of an artery. Conceptually simple, this method is difficult to implement, since blood readily clots on contact with tubing and other foreign surfaces. It was therefore a considerable achievement to have measured arterial blood pressure as long ago as 1733. After restraining a horse with ropes, the Reverend Stephen Hales inserted a goose quill into a large artery at the level of the heart so that blood could be redirected into a vertical glass tube. Within this tube, blood rose to a height of 8 feet and 3 inches above the heart, which reflects the pressure used to distribute blood around the body. The arterial pressure recorded by Hales is not representative of usual blood pressure since the horse was being restrained by ropes and would have been in considerable pain following extensive surgery without anaesthesia.

Experiments of this type allowed measurement of the blood pressure in other mammalian species. Replacing the column of blood with a column of mercury made this technique more useful. Mercury is 13.6 times heavier than water so that a column of 9 inches is sufficient for measurement of arterial blood pressure. Furthermore, a very small volume of blood is diverted into the manometer, so that measurement does not simulate haemorrhage or promote clotting. Hence, mercury manometers were used extensively for direct measurement of blood pressure in experimental animals. Use of the mercury manometer to measure pressures at which an inflatable cuff obstructs or permits arterial flow provides a method for routine measurement of arterial pressure in humans. To this end, compact instruments were devised and used routinely for clinical measurement of blood pressure in ambulant subjects or at the bedside for most of the twentieth century.

If a wide column of mercury (i.e. >5 cm) is used for measurement of blood pressure, it will be unable to detect the slight changes of pressure that accompany individual heartbeats and therefore cannot measure pulse pressure. Narrower tubes (0.5 – 1.0 cm) will detect the pressure of individual pulses but cannot be relied upon for accurate measurement. This is because oscillations caused by each pulse are superimposed upon oscillations produced by inertia of the mercury column. The periodicity of oscillations due to inertia of the mercury column is close to that of the heartbeat. Oscillations due to pulse pressure can be amplified or attenuated; hence, a narrow bore mercury manometer cannot be relied upon for measurement of pulse pressure and heartbeat frequency.

This limitation of mercury manometers is compounded by the toxicity of mercury. Mercury is very difficult to contain and very tiny amounts are released and dispersed each time a mercury manometer is used. These fine droplets of free mercury will be readily absorbed into the body on contact with skin or following inhalation. For medical and ancillary personnel who regularly use mercury manometers, progressive accumulation of free mercury is therefore inescapable. Acute toxicity arising from intermittent spillage of mercury has long been recognised as a hazard. However, containment within an enclosed space and use of forced ventilation provides adequate protection. Chronic toxicity due to escape of mercury in imperceptible amounts over long periods is much more difficult to control. As protracted low-level exposure to mercury can reduce the reproductive potential of females, use of these instruments will eventually have to be abandoned.

Toxicity can be avoided by use of a manometer that does not contain mercury. The membrane manometer is one such device and is now favoured for measurement of blood pressure. This device transmits pressure changes from arterial blood into a fluid-filled tube, capped by a thin membrane. Pressure changes arising within the tube distort the membrane proportionately. Hence, when the manometer is connected to an artery, changes of arterial pressure are followed faithfully by movements of the membrane surface. If the surface is mirrored, these tiny movements can be detected instantaneously by deflection of a beam of light. Alternatively, the relative movement with respect to a fixed surface can be measured as changed electrical capacitance. When such devices were first being developed, movements of a light beam were followed, using a scale that was placed several feet away from the manometer. Alternatively, amplifiers operating at maximum gain were used to detect capacitance changes. The complexity of these methodologies and the need for regular calibration was only acceptable for research studies. Latterly, these problems have been resolved by use of robust lasers and digital electronics. Membrane manometers are now low cost instruments with a high level of reliability. Use of such instruments has enabled self-measurement of blood pressure to become established as a precise procedure that is easy to use routinely and gives reliable results.

In anaesthetised animals, manometers are often used to monitor blood pressure continuously by connecting a pressure transducer directly to the cut end of an artery or by inserting a plastic cannula into a large artery. Corresponding measurements can be made when patients are admitted into intensive care units. Puncturing an artery is a highly invasive procedure; hence, this method is rarely used in ambulatory patients. For individuals who have high blood pressure or who are at risk of progressing to this condition, indirect measurement is preferred. Indirect measurement requires obstruction of a large artery with the aid of a pressurised cuff and continuous monitoring of pressure within the cuff during deflation. By this means it is possible to detect the onset and eventual disappearance of a pulsed pressure within the cuff. Controlled inflation and deflation of cuffs placed around the arm, wrist, or finger allow indirect measurement of blood pressure with minimal inconvenience.

2.3 What are systolic and diastolic pressures?

- Systolic blood pressure is the maximum pressure within the arterial network whilst blood is being expelled from the heart
- Diastolic blood pressure is the minimum pressure within the arterial network whilst blood is being returned to the heart

The beating mammalian heart alternates between discharging blood into arterial vessels and being refilled with blood from venous vessels. Systole is the term used to describe the phase of the pumping cycle during which the heart is discharging blood. Diastole is the term used to describe the phase of the pumping cycle during which the heart is being refilled with blood. As diastole and systole are distinct phases of each heartbeat, ejection of blood is a discontinuous process whereby a discrete bolus of blood is ejected into the arterial network at each heartbeat. Pressure within the arterial network therefore rises and falls in tandem with the heartbeat. During the ejection phase, pressure within arterial vessels rises rapidly to a maximal value that defines systolic blood pressure. During the refilling phase, valves prevent blood from returning to the heart and pressure within the major arteries declines steadily to a minimal value that defines diastolic pressure.

Because expulsion of blood is intermittent, arterial pressure must fall between heartbeats. Although substantial, this fall of pressure is cushioned by the elasticity of arterial vessels. During ejection of blood from the heart, the walls of the arterial network stretch to accommodate the increased volume of blood. Valves then close in order to isolate the arterial network whilst the heart is being refilled. As arterial vessels revert only slowly to their original dimensions, they are able to sustain a relatively high pressure within the arterial network. Hence, the difference between diastolic and systolic pressures does not exceed 40% of maximal systolic pressure.

The sudden increase of pressure that accompanies discharge of blood from the heart is disseminated as a wave along arterial vessels throughout the body. The pressure changes that produce this pulsation approximate to the pressure changes that occur within large arteries so that measurement of pulse pressures within peripheral arteries is a convenient way to define systolic and diastolic pressures. To measure these pressures, an inflatable cuff is used to obstruct blood flow into an arm (or other extremity). As pressure in the cuff is gradually reduced, the pressure at which pulsation can first be detected defines systolic pressure. As pressure within the cuff steadily declines, the arterial pulsation will strengthen and then weaken. When there is no pulsation, the pressure within the cuff defines diastolic pressure. A stethoscope is used to detect the appearance and disappearance of a pulse in an artery peripheral to the cuff when blood pressure is being measured with a mercury manometer. During oscillometric recording, the rise and fall of pulsatile pressure waves is monitored continuously within the cuff by an electronic transducer. The maximal amplitude of this oscillation defines average blood pressure and the patterns of its rise and fall allow estimation of systolic and diastolic pressures, using algorithms installed during manufacture of these instruments. Since recording, calculation and display of blood pressures are automatic, self-measurement is easy.

Semi-automatic electronic oscillometers depict blood pressures in mm of mercury. This is an accident of history. The portability and reliability of the mercury sphygmomanometer had ensured that it became a standard item within a doctor's bag and, for more than a century. When measuring blood pressure with a mercury sphygmomanometer, the vertical column of mercury has to be aligned with a calibrated scale. For convenience, blood pressures were recorded routinely in "millimetres of mercury". This unit corresponded to other metric units (cm, gm) but not to Imperial units (feet, pounds) or to more archaic measures (e.g. grains). To eliminate this diversity and to provide consistency between measurements in medicine, physics and chemistry, Standard International Units were adopted. In this unified system, pressures are expressed as Newtons per unit area (i.e. N/m^2). Since a column of mercury that is 1 millimetre high produces a pressure of 133 N/m^2, conversion from mm of mercury into Standard International Units can be achieved using a constant of proportionality. Systolic and diastolic pressures are nevertheless expressed as "mm of mercury". Such failure to adopt Standard International Units is not reasonable since introduction of digital electronic recording provided an opportunity to eliminate inconsistency with minimal effort. Ironically, semi-automatic oscillometers display pressures as "mm of mercury" even though none of these devices contain any mercury.

2.4   What is normal blood pressure?

- Measurements of usual blood pressures within developed countries spread across a wide range and no value predominates
- Arbitrarily, 140 (systolic) and 90 (diastolic) mm of mercury have been adopted as upper limits of normal pressure even though strokes and coronary heart attacks become more frequent above pressures of 115 (systolic) and 75 (diastolic) mm of mercury,
- Pressures do not exceed 100-105 (systolic) or 60-65 (diastolic) mm of mercury in non-acculturated communities, amongst whom strokes or coronary heart attacks are rare or absent

The human body has an unchanging internal environment. The characteristics of this internal environment are largely determined by automatic controls that regulate concentrations of chemicals within blood and tissue fluids. These controls becomes apparent when blood is sampled from large numbers of normal subjects, since chemical analysis will reveal that concentrations of salts, nutrients, proteins and hormones typically lie within very narrow ranges. Such automatic control is not restricted to chemicals within body fluids and extends also to some physical characteristics of the body.

Representative of this control is the constancy of body temperature, which is held at 37 °C. The importance of such close control of body temperature is revealed when skeletal muscles are cooled. Muscles shorten when groups of fibres contract in response to signals arriving at nerves that are embedded within the muscle. These fibres have a range of dimensions and lie at different distances from the brain and spinal cord. Consequently, arrival of the nerve signals has to be synchronised to ensure a smooth contraction. As transmission of signals along nerve fibres is a consequence of chemical changes, a reduction of body temperature will retard all signals. Hence, signals that have had to traverse longer distances will be delayed proportionately and will cause asynchronous contraction of the muscle. The effect of reduced temperature is perceived as clumsiness, especially in the extremities. As body temperature falls, lack of co-ordination will become increasingly obvious and ultimately the body will become immobile. Although this outcome is dramatic, restoration of normal body temperature can wholly reverse these changes.

Such close regulation of the internal environment makes many physical and chemical characteristics of the human body highly predictable. Their predictability makes it possible to use deviations from usual values as indicators of ill health. For instance, when body temperature rises above 37 °C, it is usually an indication of viral or bacterial infection. Similarly, if usual concentrations of glucose in blood exceed 1 mg per ml, this will be indicative of diabetes. It is therefore worthwhile to establish values for chemical and physical features of the body for use as standard values.

An elaborate network of reflexes operates continuously to maintain a level of blood pressure that guarantees perfusion of the brain and heart. It might be expected therefore that healthy individuals could be used to define a normal blood pressure. In some circumstances, this presumption can be valid. For instance, if blood pressures are measured in large homogenous groups of young adults (e.g. military recruits), measurements will be grouped about an averaged value. However, this averaged value will not be representative of the wider population, amongst whom a broad range of usual blood pressures is usual. In contrast to body temperature and blood glucose, measurements of blood pressure in large populations are not constrained within a narrow range and no particular value predominates.

Having a wide spread of values for a bodily characteristic that is closely controlled by reflexes is not without precedent. Body weight remains relatively constant when measured regularly over weeks or months so that weight loss can be used indicate ill health. Even so, survey of body weight within a community will reveal a wide range with no value representative for the population. Some degree of spread is to be expected since stature influences body weight. Even so, transformation into body mass index merely reduces the boundaries of the continuum. In this respect, the distribution of body mass across a population resembles the distribution of blood pressures. This close parallel is not widely recognised, possibly because the contribution of reflex controls to body mass are ignored. More usually, it is asserted that body mass is no more than a reflection of the day-to-day balance between calorific intake (as food) and loss (by exercise). This simple concept sustains a plethora of publications and TV programmes on dieting and exercise. It is likely that this attitude has retarded the development of multiple drug therapy which might be expected to provide control of body mass in the way that is closely comparable to the (now) highly effective control of blood pressure.

Surveys in developed countries reveal a broad distribution of measurements of blood pressure and of body mass. Blood pressure measurements range from <100 to >200 (systolic) and from <50 to >100 (diastolic) mm of mercury, body weights and estimates of BMI extend from <50 kg (20 kg/m^2) to >150 kg (40 kg/m^2). By way of contrast, in communities that have remained isolated and that are not yet acculturated blood pressures are very low and, like body mass, grouped within a narrow range. By our standards, individuals from these isolated communities are excessively lean since a BMI <19 kg/m^2 lies at the lower limit of BMI values in developed countries. As a corollary, we also perceive their usual blood pressures of approximately 100 (systolic) and 60 (diastolic) mm of mercury as exceptional by comparison with usual pressures in developed countries. These individuals have normal cardiovascular function and rarely, if ever, experience strokes or coronary heart disease. Their uniformly low BMI is readily understood since their diet typically requires consumption of large amounts of poorly nutritious vegetables, supplemented by occasional fruits with infrequent consumption of animal fat and protein. Why their usual blood pressure should be low and unaffected by age is not obvious. The broad spread of usual blood pressure that invariably rises with age is common to developed countries and does not indicate a plausible alternative. The link between diet and body weight by way of contrast is obvious and easily understood.

When individuals from these isolated communities adopt an urban lifestyle, their usual blood pressure becomes raised. An urban environment provides access to foods that are rich in protein and energy (e.g. tinned fish, tinned meat, bread and rice). By comparison with their former diet of fibrous roots and stalks, such foods are very palatable; hence, their calorific intake is rapidly increased and BMI rises. In the initial phase of this transformation, usual blood pressure is unaltered. However, once BMI has passed a threshold, blood pressure will rise inexorably, implying that BMI is one of the determinants of increased pressures. This "natural experiment" would be forbidden in our society –since it has the objective of making healthy subjects develop a severe illness. Observing the outcome is nevertheless decisive for it establishes that non-acculturated individuals are not protected from high blood pressure (or its untoward consequences) because of some form of intrinsic insusceptibility. Rather, their protection stems from avoidance of our lifestyle.

It is not yet certain which aspect of life in developed countries leads to susceptibility to high blood pressure. Possibly, our susceptibility stems from kidney architecture, which is fixed before birth. As expansion or regeneration of kidney tissue is not possible, a limited number of filtration units are available for urine formation. In the face of that limitation, blood pressure may be compelled to rise in order to sustain adequate levels of urine formation. High blood pressure may therefore be an inadvertent consequence of having to accommodate an inadequate filtration capacity when adults become overweight. An inadequate number of filtration units will promote use of higher filtration pressure (i.e. blood pressure) when a proportion of the filtration units will become damaged. This would reduce the rate of urine formation, causing blood pressure to rise still further in order to maintain an adequate flow of urine. Such a process could explain onset and progression of raised blood pressure as a feature of increasing body mass.

Before accepting this type of explanation for an association between high blood pressure and an urban lifestyle, it is necessary to gauge the contribution of factors unrelated to weight gain. For instance, infestation by parasites is usual in non-acculturated societies. These organisms will largely be eliminated by routine hygiene in an urban environment. This may be expected to increase body mass because of improved nutrition. As a corollary, access to sheltered dwellings as well as improved nutrition will reduce the incidence and debilitating effects of bacterial and viral infections. Set against these changes is an increased level of stress due to migration into a new culture due to loss of family infrastructure, employment uncertainties etc.. Additionally, there will be an increased risk of infection by novel agents and exposure to synthetic chemicals whose long-term effects on human health are understood poorly, if at all. In urban life, inadvertent exposure to industrial chemicals is an inescapable feature and the number of such chemicals has increased year on year. For instance, use of synthetic organic chemicals in homes and industry in USA increased from 1 billion pounds per annum in the 1940s to 400 billion pounds per annum in the 1980s. In large part, isolated communities will have avoided exposure to these chemicals, which are widely used as agrochemicals and pesticides as well as being included within foods, packaging, clothing, fuels and materials used for buildings or furnishings within an urban setting. Finally, consumption of alcohol and/or excessive amounts of salt may contribute to the changes of blood pressure that are associated with an urban lifestyle. Both substances can increase blood pressure acutely in a high proportion of individuals and it is possible that regular exposure to either of these materials may initiate or sustain processes that cause blood pressure to rise remorselessly with age.

For whatever reason, those individuals who remain within societies that are not acculturated do not experience high blood pressure. The lifestyles followed within these societies have effectively remained unchanged for many hundreds of years and might even be considered as representative of humans during prehistory. Since an urban lifestyle makes all such individuals vulnerable to development of high blood pressure, protection from high blood pressure is not an intrinsic characteristic of these individuals. On balance, it seems more likely that high blood pressure is an untoward consequence of a changed diet and/or increased body mass. It is possible that this type of explanation may extend to other major health changes that arise when transferring to an urban lifestyle (See Table 2).

Factor	Preliterate communities	Urban communities	Incidence of increased risk
Salt intake (mmol/day)	1	120-210	100%
Body mass index (kg/m²)	< 20	> 27	>90% by sixth decade
Systolic pressure (mm of mercury)	100	> 140	>95% by sixth decade
Serum cholesterol (mmol)	3.2	6.0	>99% by sixth decade
Death from stroke or heart attack	Rare or absent	Epidemic (from fifth decade onwards)	>1.2 % per annum
Death from second stroke or coronary heart attack	Not applicable	Epidemic	>5% per annum
Diabetes/pre-diabetes	Rare or absent	Epidemic	40%
Asthma/allergy	Rare or absent	Epidemic	30-40%

Table 2. Contribution of urban lifestyle to chronic illnesses

Preliterate communities are living relicts of earlier societies whose members might reasonably be considered to have blood pressures that are representative for our species. Comparable measurements are not available for feral primates, excepting for baboons whose averaged pressures of 114 (systolic) and 64 (diastolic) mm of mercury are not far removed from usual pressures of 100 (systolic) and 60 (diastolic) mm of mercury that can be cited for non-acculturated humans. Populations of humans that have experienced severe reduction of food intake due to warfare or famine also have lowered blood pressure. For instance, survey of pressures in starving populations from the highlands of Ethiopia revealed pressures between 106 and 109 (systolic) and between 73 and 75 (diastolic) mm of mercury, irrespective of age. As in non-acculturated populations, such individuals are exceptionally slim, with a BMI that averages 19 kg/m². It is tempting to conclude that blood pressures are low in these populations as a direct consequence of restricted food intake since adults with a body mass index as low as 19 kg/m² are infrequent within developed countries. Whether low blood pressure stems solely from loss of body weight must be considered unproven since contributions from increased vulnerability to infections, changed gut flora and infestation by parasites have yet to be excluded.

It has been possible to investigate the connection between increased body weight and increased blood pressure by monitoring young West African men as they move into an urban environment. On leaving their rural villages to enter an urban environment, they reduce overall physical activity and increase their intake of food. Once their BMI exceeds 21.5 kg/m², they become predisposed to raised blood pressure. In developed countries, a BMI in excess of 21.5 kg/m² is commonplace and >90% of adults of West African origin who are resident within USA will have a BMI >21.5 kg/m². Attempting to define normal blood pressure by survey of these individuals would not be appropriate and attempting to define normal blood pressure in comparable ethnic groups are likely to be equally unrewarding. Measuring usual blood pressures in populations within developed countries has merit as an aid to improved healthcare. However, these measurements cannot be used to define normal blood pressure.

Given this impasse, it has been necessary to devise an alternative method to recognise normal blood pressure. It is well established that the frequency of strokes and coronary heart attacks is directly proportional to blood pressure over a wide range of pressures. Hence, it can be inferred that blood pressure will be normal when reduction of usual blood pressure does not influence the risk of strokes and heart attacks. The frequency of strokes and coronary heart attacks will increase in direct proportion to increased blood pressure for pressures that are in excess of 115 (systolic) and 75 (diastolic) mm of mercury. Below these pressures there is a residual increased risk that cannot be predicted from the usual blood pressure. In preliterate, non-acculturated communities, blood pressures are even lower but whether pressures of 100 (systolic) and 60 (diastolic) mm of mercury could, or should, provide benchmarks for normal blood pressure is debatable. It is not possible to test directly whether these pressures increase the risk of strokes and coronary heart attacks in subjects who are living in developed countries. Such low levels are relatively infrequent. Furthermore, previous exposure to raised blood pressure, deposition of cholesterol in arterial walls and loss of filtration units in the kidney would have to be excluded as sources of vulnerability to strokes and coronary heart attacks. Ascertaining whether blood pressures that are usual in non-acculturated communities could eliminate strokes and coronary heart attacks in developed countries would require large prospective studies that would be very expensive. Even so, clarification of this issue is important since total avoidance of strokes and coronary heart attacks has implications beyond the technical issue of setting a valid level for normal blood pressure. If regular monitoring of blood pressure in adults from an early age could substantially diminished the frequency of strokes and heart attacks in later life, it would considerably increase life expectancy and have major implications for provision of overall heath care.

When arterial vessels have been damaged by high pressure, strokes and coronary heart attacks become more frequent. The uncertain location and general inaccessibility of damaged vessels usually precludes measurement of damage to individual arteries. Methods that might be used for measuring such damage are technically exacting and require customised instruments. The retina, which can be examined routinely with an ophthalmoscope, provides an exception. Even so, repeated measurements are impractical when large numbers of patients have to be monitored over long periods. By way of contrast, self-measurement of blood pressure as an indicator of overall arterial damage is relatively straightforward, easily repeated and can be correlated retrospectively with instances of death or disability due to a stroke or a coronary heart attack.

Sustained exposure of arterial vessels to high blood pressure makes them increasingly vulnerable to rupture or obstruction. If either event occurs within the brain or heart, a stroke or a coronary heart attack will follow. Strokes and coronary heart attacks can be recognised with some certainty from clinical symptoms and will have been reported in medical case notes or recorded on death certificates. Hence, the frequency of strokes and coronary heart attacks can be defined with considerable certainty, even over many years. By estimating the frequency of strokes or coronary heart attacks in subjects whose blood pressure is being measured routinely, it can be shown that the risk of either misfortune is directly proportional to usual blood pressure (See Tables 3 & 4). Measuring the frequency of these events therefore provides a simple index of overall damage to blood vessels resulting from increased blood pressure.

Age	Systolic pressure (mm of mercury)			
	120	140	160	180
40s	<1	<1	<1	<1
50s	1	3	8	20
60s	3	8	20	35
70s	15	25	50	100
80s	50	90	140	200

Table 3. Risk of death (fold increase) from a stroke rises both with age (decade of life) and with systolic pressure measured whilst at rest

Age	Systolic pressure (mm of mercury)			
	120	140	160	180
40s	1	3	5	11
50s	4	7	15	30
60s	11	20	30	60
70s	25	50	75	120
80s	70	110	180	250

Table 4. Risk of death (fold increase) from a coronary heart attack rises both with age (decade of life) and with systolic pressure measured whilst at rest

The relationship between increased blood pressure and corresponding damage that arises in organs other than the heart and the brain has not been studied as exhaustively, but available information indicates that raised blood pressure is similarly predictive of damage to vision and to the kidneys.

When usual blood pressure exceeds 140 (systolic) or 90 (diastolic) mm of mercury, the risk of strokes and coronary heart attacks is increased substantially. It is therefore easy to justify using these pressure levels for diagnosis of high blood pressure and for using drugs to lower blood pressure. Attempting to use this approach for definition of normal levels of pressure is not straightforward. The incidence of strokes or coronary heart attacks at high levels of blood pressure is quite clearly increased. At lower pressures, the incidence of these events becomes progressively more difficult to define. This is because strokes and coronary heart attacks occur infrequently when individuals have pre-hypertension and become even less frequent when pressures approach levels that might be considered normal. Hence, exceptionally large numbers of subjects are needed to detect these low rates. So many subjects would have to be monitored that the resources of any single research group would be overwhelmed. Hence, to obtain reliable estimates of risk at pressures below 140 (systolic) or 90 (diastolic) mm of mercury has required amalgamation of results from many studies. By combining 61 separate studies, it has been possible to assemble results that report on outcomes during 12.7 million patient-years. Amongst the one million participants (aged between 40 and 89 years) recruited into these studies, approximately 12,000 died from strokes, 34,000 died from coronary heart disease and there were 10,000 deaths from other vascular diseases. An absence of pre-existing vascular disease was a precondition for recruitment into these studies. Yet there were 56,000 deaths from vascular disease, a frequency that almost matches the 66,000 deaths attributed to all other causes. This high frequency of death from vascular disease is consistent with the projection by the World Health Organisation that vascular diseases will be the predominant cause of death in developed countries by 2020.

Within these large populations, the risk of death from vascular disease is predicted by usual blood pressure (See Figures 2, 3 & 4). Predictions are similar whether systolic or diastolic pressures are used as indicators, although the average from these two pressures (mid-blood pressure) is the most reliable predictor of death from stroke or coronary heart disease (See Figure 5). Individuals who are aged between 40 and 69 have a risk of death from strokes, coronary heart disease that is doubled by an increase of pressure of 20 (systolic) or 10 (diastolic) mm of mercury. This increased risk is cumulative for systolic pressures between 115 and 195 mm of mercury. Hence, the risk of stroke will double whether systolic blood pressure rises from 115 to 135, from 135 to 155, from 155 to 175 or from 175 to 195 mm of mercury. It follows that increasing systolic pressure from 115 mm to 195 mm of mercury would increase the risk of a stroke or a coronary heart attack by eight-fold (i.e. 800%). Even though the increased risk due to raised blood pressure can now be specified with some certainty, the problem of defining level for no increased risk has yet to be resolved. At present, the only certain conclusion to be drawn from survival data is that ill health due to damaged arterial vessels is increased if blood pressures exceed 115 (systolic) or 75 (diastolic) mm of mercury.

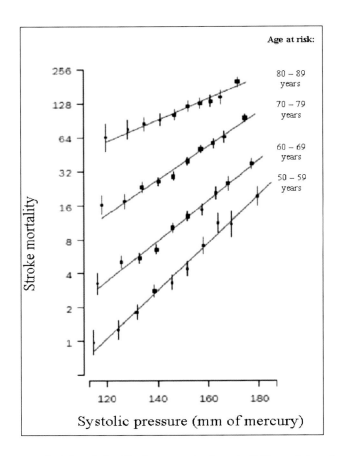

Figure 2. Increased risk of death from a stroke at different levels of blood pressure in each decade of life

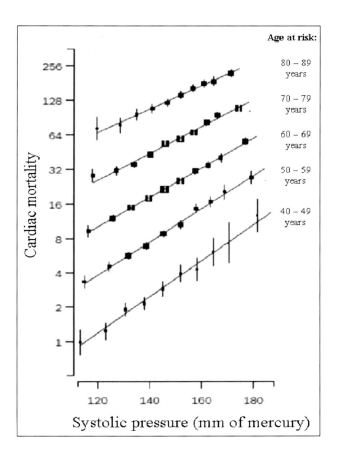

Figure 3. Increased risk of death from a coronary heart attack at different levels of blood pressure in each decade of life

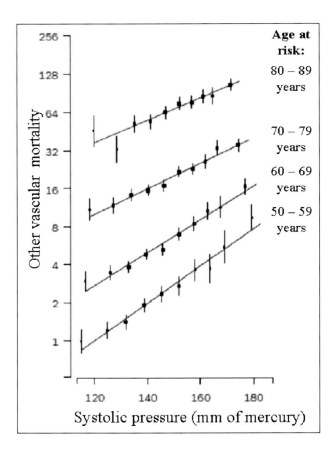

Figure 4. Increased risk of death from a vascular disease other than strokes or coronary heart attacks at different levels of blood pressure in each decade of life

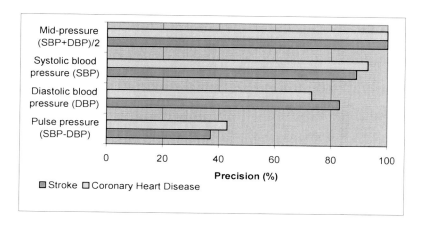

Figure 5. Precision of prediction of mortality due to strokes or heart attacks from systolic pressure (SBP), diastolic pressure (DBP), mid-pressure (SBP/2+DBP/2) and pulse pressure (SBP-DPB)

2.5   What causes high blood pressure?

- Malfunction of regulatory systems that prevent a fall of blood pressure can cause pressure to rise inappropriately
- Pressures may rise because of increased responsiveness to materials that constrict arterial muscle and/or increased release of such materials
- Pressures may rise if there is decreased responsiveness to materials that relax arterial muscle and/or decreased release of such materials
- Pressures may rise when blood volume is not controlled
- In developed countries, onset of high blood pressure may be linked to increased food intake and reduced physical activity

In certain circumstances, onset of high blood pressure can be anticipated. Pregnancy is the most obvious example since raised blood pressure is likely to occur in more than 30% of first pregnancies. High blood pressure is also a well-recognised characteristic of specific diseases. For instance, narrowing of the renal artery (renal stenosis) or proliferation of cysts within the kidney (polycystic kidney) will reduce blood flow into the kidney and thereby produce increased blood pressure. For the kidney, any reduction of inflow will mimic the reduction of perfusion that occurs during haemorrhage. Being unable to differentiate reduction of renal blood flow due to haemorrhage from a selective reduction due to narrowing of the renal artery, the kidney releases renin in both circumstances. On contact with blood, this enzyme will detach a small peptide that can produce an impressive rise of blood pressure.

Initially, this small peptide was referred to jointly as "angiotonin" or "hypertensin". To eliminate confusion, these terms were eventually melded into "angiotensin". On injection into normal animals, purified angiotensin produced a striking increase of blood pressure and was considerably more potent than other naturally occurring substances. It was therefore confidently anticipated that the blood of patients with high blood pressure would contain increased amounts of angiotensin. Certainly, the amount is increased but these concentrations are nevertheless insufficient to contract human arterial muscle. Hence, if the onset and maintenance of high blood pressure are to be explained by overproduction of angiotensin, effects other than direct contraction of arterial muscle have to be identified.

This issue was resolved by demonstration of two further properties of angiotensin. Firstly, and quite unexpectedly, it was demonstrated that angiotensin is a potent stimulus for secretion of aldosterone. Aldosterone is a hormone that is secreted from the adrenal gland to ensure that loss of sodium into urine is minimal. The sodium ions that are retained within the body remain in the blood and, by abstracting water from surrounding tissues, they increase the total volume of plasma within the circulation. This increased volume compels arterial vessels to expand and the increased tension within their elastic wall manifests as raised blood pressure. A second unexpected property of angiotensin is the activation of a specialised population of nerve cells at the base of the brain. Nerve fibres emerging from these cells ramify throughout the body. On being activated by angiotensin, these nerve fibres contract arterial muscles, which causes blood pressure to rise. Having established these additional properties, it is reasonable to expect that high blood pressure could arise because there is formation of angiotensin when the flow of blood into the kidneys was reduced. The existence of this specific mechanism does not preclude other mechanisms that could produce raised blood pressure without involvement of the kidney.

Any fall in blood pressure will immediately initiate reflex responses throughout the body. Such responses restore usual blood pressure and guarantee adequate blood flow into the brain and heart. Concurrent use of several independent reflexes to achieve this objective is advantageous for each reflex provides a safeguard against a large fall of blood pressure that could be lethal. Even so, there is an inherent disadvantage in having a multiplicity of reflex controls since the chance of malfunction increases with the number of separate controls. Such malfunction is a hazard because, unlike a fall in blood pressure, raised blood pressure is not an immediate threat to well being. There is therefore no urgent need to counter raised blood pressure automatically even though prolonged high blood pressure will ultimately produce ill health. It will be obvious that dysfunction could affect any one of a number of distinct control systems. Hence, when considering the treatment of high blood pressure, it is inappropriate to focus upon a particular local hormone as the pivotal control mechanism. Nevertheless, over the years, excessive formation and release of adrenaline, nor-adrenaline, renin, angiotensin I, angiotensin II, endothelin and aldosterone have separately enjoyed periods of popularity.

There is no obvious reason for placement of a particular chemical as a pivotal mediator of high blood pressure. Any of the local hormones so far implicated in blood pressure control might participate in the elevation of blood pressure. For instance, release of adrenaline from adrenal glands and from sympathetic nerve endings will increase the strength and frequency of the heartbeat and cardiac output. Adrenaline will also raise blood pressure by constriction of arterial muscle but as it relaxes arterial muscle in some tissues, the net effect is an attenuation of the increased pressure that results from an increased output of blood from the heart. Nor-adrenaline is released concurrently with adrenaline from the bulbous endings of sympathetic nerves in arterial vessels. By constricting small arteries throughout the body, nor-adrenaline produces a marked rise of blood pressure. By way of contrast, renin is secreted from cells in the kidney and affects blood pressure indirectly by promoting secretion of aldosterone from the adrenal gland. By effecting a retention of sodium, this hormone increases the total volume of blood and hence raises pressure. Unexpectedly, the ability of angiotensin to contract arterial muscle does not determine its role in blood pressure control even though it is 40 times more potent than adrenaline as a stimulus of arterial constriction. This surprising outcome indicates that vasoconstrictor local hormones or nerve transmitter substances need not necessarily merit special attention because of their potency. For instance, vasopressin and thromboxanes are vasoconstrictor substances whose potency in producing contraction of arterial muscle is readily countered by release into circulating blood of a variety of vasodilator materials, including adrenaline, dopamine, adenosine, bradykinin, and other peptides. Atrial natiuretic peptide is one such relaxant and merits attention because it has the additional property of being able to contribute to blood volume control. This substance is released from the wall of the heart and, in addition to producing a relaxation of arterial muscle, counters expansion of blood volume by promoting secretion of sodium ions into urine. The lining cells of arterial vessels are able to cause comparable relaxation of arterial muscle by secreting nitric oxide locally. Because of its localised formation, nitric oxide is increasingly viewed as an intermediary that could determine relaxation of arterial muscle in a wide range of circumstances. The potent vasoconstrictor peptide endothelin could have an analogous role by producing localised contraction of arterial muscle. If there is overproduction or increased sensitivity to a material that is central to contraction of arterial muscle (e.g. endothelin), the resulting imbalance could underlie high blood pressure. Equally, this form of imbalance might stem from decreased formation or diminished sensitivity to an agent that is central to relaxation of arterial muscle (e.g. nitric oxide).

Coexistence of several independent mechanisms for producing increased blood pressure is a "belt and braces strategy " that avoids life-threatening reduction of blood pressure should one control system become ineffective. For instance, although the kidney plays a major role in blood pressure regulation, it is possible for the body to accommodate loss of both kidneys. A practical consequence of this multiplicity of controls is that drugs can be devised to act selectively upon specific control mechanisms. For instance, beta blockers were devised to oppose some of the effects of adrenaline and nor-adrenaline; ACE inhibitors were selected to suppress activation of enzymes that convert angiotensin I into angiotensin II; diuretics were selected to suppress transportation of specific ions during formation of urine within kidney tubules. Because of their distinctive effects, these drugs can be used in combination and, as their actions are independent one from another, they should produce effects that are additive. For some combinations, interaction is synergistic and the fall of pressure will be exaggerated. A further advantage using these drugs in combination to lower blood pressure is that side effects will be minimised.

The ability of drug categories to achieve greater effectiveness when used in combination reinforces the conclusion that no singular control defect determines high blood pressure. Even so, it does not exclude entirely the possibility of some universal "cause of high blood pressure". For instance, structural changes in the muscular layer of small arteries could provide such a unifying mechanism. The sustained stresses that arise in the vessel wall when there is prolonged elevation of blood pressure serves as a stimulus for enlargement of arterial muscle. It seems self-evident that strengthening of arterial muscle in response to increased pressure should be inherently protective. However, such a change becomes counterproductive when the expanding muscular layer is thrown into folds by the unyielding fibrous coat that envelops arterial vessels. These folds obstruct the flow of blood and cause blood pressure to rise by a mechanism that is unrelated to physiological control and that is not amenable to control by drugs.

The increased resistance to flow that results from enlargement of arterial muscle will be intensified if the processes that limit muscular contraction become compromised. Continuous formation of nitric oxide by cells that line the inner surface of healthy vessels controls relaxation of arterial muscle. When arterial muscle expands and is thrown into folds and bulges, the smooth flow of blood along the inner surface of arterial vessels will be disrupted. Resulting turbulence will damage the lining cells and diminishes their capacity to generate nitric oxide. Such a reduction of nitric oxide formation occurs when deposits of cholesterol distort the vessel wall and produce turbulent flow. In these circumstances, the rate of formation of nitric oxide may be insufficient to counter arterial constriction and will promote raised blood pressure. For this reason it can be anticipated that using statins to reduce cholesterol deposition will help to suppress high blood pressure, even though these drugs have no direct effect on the heart, arterial muscle or on processes that control blood volume.

Physiological control of blood pressure is influenced by extrinsic factors, such as diet or regular exercise. Making comparisons between groups of patients can reveal the effect of such factors. For instance, such comparison will detect an association between the severity of high blood pressure and the averaged daily intake of salt or of alcohol. A similar association is evident for intake of energy-rich food and of cholesterol. Comparisons of this type have been used to demonstrate that certain lifestyles favour an earlier onset and increased severity of high blood pressure. As a corollary, it is possible to use this approach to detect whether there is a significant reduction of blood pressure when lifestyle is changed. For instance, usual blood pressure can be lowered by reducing the daily intake of sodium (by avoiding processed foods), by increasing the daily intake of potassium (by eating greater quantities of fruit and vegetables) or of nitrate (by eating certain vegetables). Similarly, regular consumption of garlic or of oily fish and regular participation in aerobic exercise will produce net reductions of blood pressure. Even so, not all lifestyle changes influence blood pressure. For instance, neither taking up, nor stopping, smoking has a direct effect upon blood pressure. Of the various associations detected, the linkage between high blood pressure and the "metabolic disease" is possibly the most important. Metabolic disease is characterised by increased abdominal girth (>102 mm for men and 88 mm for women) coupled with high blood pressure, impaired glucose tolerance, raised concentrations of triglycerides in blood, a decreased concentration of HDL-cholesterol in blood and a resistance to the metabolic effects of insulin. Metabolic disease is now prevalent in developed countries and, at the turn of the century, there were 47 million such individuals in the USA. The incidence of this disease continues to rise; hence, it is to be expected that metabolic disease will drive up the incidence of high blood pressure in developed countries. Given this situation, it is can be anticipated that lethal events precipitated by high blood pressure will inevitably predominate as a cause of death in developed countries.

2.6   What are the consequences of high blood pressure?

- By damaging the arterial wall, sustained high blood pressure increases the risk of obstruction
- In the brain, impaired perfusion will predispose to dementia as well as causing transient ischaemic attacks or strokes
- In the heart, impaired perfusion manifests as angina and localised blockage will cause a coronary heart attack
- Malfunction of the heart induces left ventricle enlargement, atrial fibrillation, ventricular arrhythmia and congestive heart failure
- In the kidney, there is a reduced rate of urine formation and damage to filtration units causes microalbuminuria and proteinuria
- Raised blood pressure can increase the risk of stroke or coronary heart attack by >20-fold

Asthmatics experience episodic breathlessness that is associated with tightness in the chest and a reduced intake of air. These symptoms occur because muscles in the asthmatic airways are enlarged and excessively responsive to activation by physiological or pathological stimuli. To ameliorate these symptoms, drugs have been developed that relax airway muscles selectively. Asthmatics perceive the onset of airway obstruction as a tightening in the chest and are able to self-administer drugs as a fine mist from an inhaler to relieve symptoms. Such treatment will usually provide adequate control of symptoms and admission to hospital is infrequent. Even intense contraction of airway muscles infrequently leads to death.

Enlargement of arterial muscle in high blood pressure is difficult to distinguish from the enlargement of airway muscle in asthma. Yet activation of enlarged muscles in the arterial wall has a markedly dissimilar outcome. Contraction of airway muscle leads to attacks of asthma by reducing ventilation. Contraction of arterial muscle to produce raised blood pressure does not markedly change the flow rate through arteries. Hence, whereas contraction of airway muscles produces the discomforting symptoms of asthma, contraction of arterial muscle during high blood pressure is without symptoms.

Despite this lack of symptoms, high blood pressure is relentless in causing damage to arterial vessels. Such changes are slow to develop and are more likely to arise when exposure to high pressures is sustained over long periods. Damage is cumulative and can unexpectedly manifest as sudden malfunction of a vital organ. Consequently, deaths from high blood pressure are relatively frequent and often occur when individuals are not receiving medical care. In these respects, deaths due to high blood pressure differ from deaths due to asthma, which typically occur whilst patients are being treated, often when under intensive care.

Raised blood pressure is not invariably pathological and, especially in early life, it is likely to be a physiological response to intense physical activity (e.g. fighting, running etc.). Exposure to such transient increased pressure does not damage healthy arteries. Instead, it is the protracted exposure to raised pressure that causes damage by initiating irreversible structural changes in arteries. The intensity and duration of exposure needed to produce structural damage is a matter for conjecture. Pregnancy provides a natural experiment that gives some indication as to how long vessels may tolerate increased pressure without causing structural changes. It is likely that there is little arterial damage since the high blood pressure of pregnancy typically resolves within 24 hours of termination, although the risk of stroke in later life is approximately doubled. It is possible that biochemical changes in pregnancy protect arterial vessels from lasting damage. More probably there is a need for exposure to excessive pressures over many months or even years if changes are to be irreversible.

Within the brain, heart, eye or kidney the consequences of arterial damage are severe. Strokes or coronary heart attacks are sudden calamitous events that can be life threatening. The arterial damage that leads to impaired vision and kidney failure has a more insidious onset but the consequences are no less important. Monitoring the onset, or outcome, of such illnesses provides a simple and convenient measure of the consequences of prolonged high blood pressure. By use of surveys, the risk of experiencing a stroke, a coronary heart attack or other vascular disease can now readily be predicted by measurement of usual blood pressure (See Figures 2, 3 & 4). It is noteworthy that the increased risk stemming from raised blood pressure becomes apparent during the fourth decade of life for coronary heart attacks and during the fifth decade for strokes (See Figures 6 & 7).

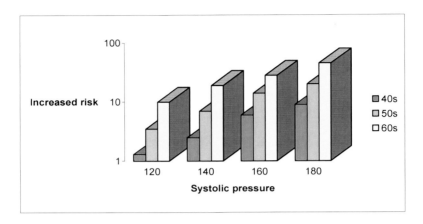

Figure 6. Increased risk of death from coronary heart attack due to raised systolic blood pressure during the fourth, fifth and sixth decades of life.

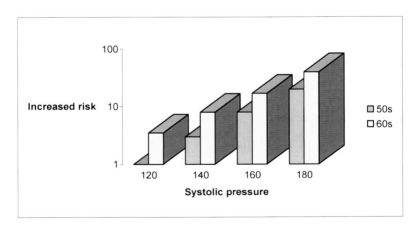

Figure 7. Increased risk of death from stroke due to raised systolic blood pressure in the fifth and sixth decades of life.

Arterial vessels that have been damaged by prolonged exposure to high blood pressure are vulnerable to damage when there are sudden surges of pressure.

Although a thickening of arterial muscle will strengthen the vessel wall, asymmetrical enlargement is a source of stresses that increase the chance of fissures appearing within the vessel wall. Fragments of tissue and clotted material will detach more readily from such sites. This is hazardous because such material will lodge downstream and may cause protracted loss of flow when accumulation of white blood cells and local activation of the clotting process amplify physical blockade.

When arteries are blocked, the effect of localised loss of blood flow depends upon the tissue affected. Within skeletal muscle, arteries form a network whose interconnections permit re-routing of blood flow. Hence, despite the sudden discomfort of severe cramp, there may be no significant long-term damage to skeletal muscle. Those tissues that need a constant supply of oxygen and that lack the facility of diversion of flow will be especially vulnerable. For instance, irreversible damage will arise within minutes of blockade in a small artery within the brain and can cause dysfunction that seems disproportionate when fibres from affected nerve cells extend to the periphery. As in skeletal muscle, localised loss of flow will produce pain in heart muscle but, as rest is not possible, recovery is more difficult. As for brain, damage in the heart can be disproportionate. For instance, if specialised cells that synchronise contraction of heart muscle receive inadequate amounts of oxygen, pumping efficiency of the heart will be compromised. In tissues other than the brain and heart, damage may occur, yet can remain unnoticed. For instance, when plasma escapes from arterial vessels in the retina, "cotton wool spots" appear on the retina. Although not painful, these areas of repair will compromise vision by obstructing transmission of light to the underlying retina. In the kidneys, incremental arterial damage results in successive elimination of filtration units that initiate urine formation. Such damage may remain undetected until urine formation is reduced sufficiently to indicate kidney failure.

Peaks of systolic pressure experienced by patients with high blood pressure are, on average, higher than those experienced by subjects with normal blood pressure. Even so, such pulses of high pressure should not pose a problem since it is normal for arteries to experience brief pulses of high pressure during physical exertion. However, if the vessel wall has been damaged already by exposure to high blood pressure, pulses of high pressure may extend the area of damage. Sites of turbulent flow are especially vulnerable since damage to the vessel lining, will enable plasma to accumulate within the vessel wall. Sequestered plasma provides a focus for local accumulation of platelets and white cells. On entering the vessel wall these white cells ingest the accumulated albumin as well as clotted blood, immune complexes and lipids such as cholesterol. If not metabolised within these cells, such materials will be deposited locally. Deposited material will not be distributed uniformly and, when the arterial wall is stretched, stresses will arise at the boundaries of these asymmetric deposits. The fissures that eventually appear will be widened and deepened by successive peaks of systolic pressure and serve as sites for activation of the clotting cascade.

Physiological clotting occurs only when vessels are torn or severed. At the site of damage, platelets will clump together and secrete substances that strongly contract arterial muscle. The consequent reduction of blood flow allows congealed blood to collect and become transformed into a more permanent barrier. Clumping of platelets or coagulation of plasma proteins within intact arteries would disrupt the smooth flow of blood. To guard against any inappropriate accumulation of platelets, cells that line the inner surface of arteries continuously secrete substances that suppress activation of platelets. This inhibitory effect is diminished when lining cells become damaged, as at sites of turbulent flow. This causes platelets to adhere to the vessel lining and, as white cells accumulate, they will serve as a focus for localised coagulation. These masses of clotted blood prevent flow of blood as they grow or break up to impact downstream within narrower vessels. Both types of blockage will restrict delivery of oxygen and nutrients to tissues. The consequences of blockade by clotted blood are difficult to distinguish from the effects of arterial rupture. Differentiation is important nonetheless, since therapeutic measures that disrupt clotted blood would increase the loss of blood if a vessel wall has been breached.

There is a seamless progression from pre-hypertension into hypertension. Both phases of this disease lack clinical symptoms and damage to target organs can only be detected by clinical or laboratory tests. For instance, the rate of filtration of blood within the kidney may be reduced and protein may be detectable in urine; the left ventricle of the heart may have become enlarged;

retinal damage may be evident and there may be reduced blood flow into the white matter of the brain as a forerunner of dementia. If high blood pressure remains undetected or is not treated, damage to these target organs will progress until clinical symptoms become evident, including chronic renal failure, angina, reduced cardiac output, arrhythmia, dementia and transient attacks of brain ischaemia. Eventually, damage to these organs will lead to end-stage diseases that include total renal failure and congestive heart failure in addition to strokes and coronary heart attacks (See Figure 8).

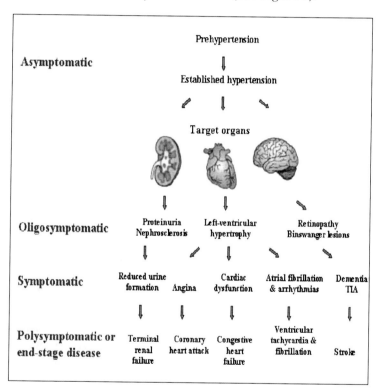

Figure 8. Early detection and treatment of high blood pressure is needed to prevent cumulative damage to target organs .

2.7 Cholesterol and high blood pressure

- When plasma concentrations are high cholesterol is likely to enter the arterial wall
- Deposits of cholesterol decrease elasticity and damage the lining of arteries by inducing turbulent flow
- Exuded plasma attracts phagocytes which metabolise or deport cholesterol
- Phagocytes that become resident promote the growth of arterial muscle
- Overgrowth of arterial muscle increases the resistance to flow in small arteries, leading to increased blood pressure
- Sequestered cholesterol reduces the ability of small arteries to relax by suppressing formation and actions of nitric oxide

Sequestration of cholesterol within arterial vessels is a characteristic feature of arteriosclerosis. The resulting inflammatory changes cause flexible elastic fibres to be replaced by materials that are inelastic. This change is often described as hardening of the arteries and vessels that are stiffened in this way do not adequately cushion pressure surges. This inability to dissipate stress is most pronounced when there is asymmetric deposition of cholesterol. Such shearing stresses favour the development of fissures and these may deepen sufficiently to extend across the full thickness of the vessel wall. Fissures provide sites for inappropriate activation of the clotting cascade and are vulnerable to damage during surges of high pressure. This increases the risk of heart attack or stroke whenever blood pressure is raised. For instance, men who are 50 years old men and have blood pressure of 160 (systolic) or 110 (diastolic) mm of mercury, the risk of a stroke or coronary heart attack is between 0.5 and 1% over a one-year period. This risk is doubled when there is a large amount of cholesterol in circulating blood.

Arteriosclerosis may be viewed as an inappropriate reaction of the body to an excessive burden of cholesterol. Yet arteriosclerosis cannot be arrested or prevented simply by excluding cholesterol from our diet. Cholesterol is an essential component of all cell membranes and is a precursor for synthesis of steroids and bile constituents. It is absorbed from the gut as a component of animal fats (e.g. beef and mutton fat). Being an essential constituent of all cell membranes, cholesterol must be present in adequate amounts for use in tissue repair. The body cannot rely upon diet alone for this material and, if dietary intake is insufficient, cholesterol will be synthesised from fat stores within the liver. Whether absorbed from the gut or synthesised by the liver, cholesterol circulates in blood to ensure prompt delivery to tissues that are growing or being repaired. To aid delivery, cholesterol is attached to lipoproteins. For synthesis of new cell membranes, cholesterol is attached to a low-density lipoprotein (LDL). For transportation away from sites of tissue breakdown, cholesterol is attached to a high-density lipoprotein (HDL). In large part, cholesterol circulates while attached to HDL and is recycled within the liver. However, as synthesis of new cell membranes has an over-riding priority, other specialised proteins can be used to transfer cholesterol between HDL and LDL.

Because dietary cholesterol is supplemented by cholesterol that has been synthesised within the liver, LDL-cholesterol circulates in amounts that are adequate for metabolic needs. However, if consumption of animal fats is excessive, circulating LDL-cholesterol will become super abundant. In this circumstance, LDL-cholesterol is liable to pose a problem whenever the arterial wall is injured, as following physical or chemical damage, infections or immunological reactions. Such injuries cause the relatively impermeable arterial wall to become porous. This increased porosity enables cholesterol and other plasma constituents to traverse the inner lining and accumulate within the vessel wall. Accumulation of plasma during injury to skin, muscle or joints will produce a turgid swelling. No such swelling can arise in arteries because they have an inflexible sheath. Consequently, plasma is retained at the site of injury.

Processes such as localised infection and deposition of immune complexes can damage the lining of small arteries. However, it is the continuous damage that accompanies turbulence that most obviously favours arteriosclerosis at particular anatomical sites. The slight damage produced by turbulence of flowing blood is sufficient to produce a sustained inflammatory reaction. As a result, the porosity of the inner lining of small arteries is increased and cholesterol will accumulate. Turbulence is exaggerated whenever there is a diversion of blood flow, as at arterial bifurcations or wherever bulges and folds of proliferating arterial muscle disrupt flow. Such turbulence is intensified by elevated blood pressure. Hence, areas of arteriosclerosis will expand more rapidly whenever high blood pressure is poorly controlled and whenever large amounts of cholesterol are present in the circulation.

Plasma that has accumulated within the arterial wall attracts white blood cells from circulating blood. After attaching to the arterial lining, these cells transform into macrophages, which are phagocytic cells that roam around the site of damage and ingest droplets of tissue fluid in a manner that closely resembles the feeding activities of an amoeba in pond water. These macrophages are able to degrade many of the components of accumulated plasma and will store any material that cannot be digested. After elimination of accumulated plasma, macrophages will usually disperse before dying. However, if increased porosity of the vessel wall is sustained, pre-programmed death can become deferred and the phagocytes become permanent residents. Resident macrophages continue to ingest and degrade materials for as long as the process of plasma accumulation continues.

Cholesterol is one of many plasma constituents that can be metabolised by phagocytic cells. However, if large quantities of cholesterol are present in plasma, the metabolic capacity of these cells can be overwhelmed. When this occurs, increasing numbers of cholesterol-rich droplets will accumulate within their cytoplasm. These engorged macrophages can be readily visualised by using dyes that partition into fats. Under the microscope, the content of these engorged cells has the appearance of foam and these "foam cells" accumulate on, or beneath, the lining of arterial vessel walls. "Fatty streaks" that are comprised of such cells provide a foundation for cholesterol deposition. Over time, deposits will enlarge and become consolidated into "plaques of atheroma" which comprise masses of cholesterol mixed with tissue debris. Fatty streaks arise because macrophages are unable to metabolise excessive amounts of cholesterol. Hence, such deposits appear earlier and grow more rapidly if consumption of cholesterol is excessive or if individuals are genetically predisposed to retain excessive amounts of cholesterol in blood. Alternatively or additionally, regular use of certain drugs (notably steroids) or regular inhalation of tobacco smoke will accelerate accumulation of cholesterol.

If the concentration of LDL-cholesterol in plasma can be reduced, accumulation of cholesterol may be arrested and some of the deposited cholesterol may be transported away from the vessel wall. This type of process accounts for the paucity of fatty streaks in individuals who have been malnourished for long periods. It also explains why patients with partial obstruction of coronary arteries can experience increased coronary blood flow by a near-complete elimination of cholesterol from their diet. Statins are drugs that were developed to reduce formation of cholesterol and, by analogy with dietary depletion, were expected to retard progression of arteriosclerosis in obstructed vessels. A reduced frequency of coronary heart attacks when these drugs are used as a preventive therapy accords with such expectation. The greater protection achieved when higher doses are used routinely implies that obstruction may be reversed, as well as arrested, by treatment with this category of drugs.

Although cholesterol can be returned into the circulation from sites of deposition, other consequences of this type of inflammation can only be reversed with difficulty, if at all. This is because local hormones that are released from sequestered macrophages stimulate proliferation and growth of arterial muscle. In arterial vessels that have been severely damaged, as following physical injury, such localised promotion of muscle growth is necessary to ensure structural integrity of repaired tissue. For less severe injury, proliferation of arterial muscle is unwarranted. Thus, modest inflammatory reaction at sites of turbulent blood flow would not normally induce overgrowth of arterial muscle. Only if the concentrations of LDL-cholesterol in blood are raised will this aberrant reaction occur at sites of turbulent flow. In that circumstance, accumulated plasma will attract macrophages and these cells will promote growth of arterial muscle by generating local hormones. Because the fibrous sheath that encases arteries remains undamaged, enlargement causes the muscles to be thrown into folds that disrupt the smooth flow of blood and produce turbulence. These folds will subsequently serve as a focus for further damage, leading to a progressive accumulation of cholesterol. Over time these deposits will become organised into rigid plaques that are analogous to scars or scabs on the skin.

Clinical symptoms of arteriosclerosis arise when the flow of blood through arteries is insufficient for metabolic needs. For instance, when blood flow into leg muscles is restricted by arteriosclerosis, the speed and duration of walking will be diminished by painful cramp. A comparable limitation to the blood supply of heart muscle will produce the disabling chest pain of angina during exertion. As well as producing chronic functional changes by reducing blood flow, arteriosclerosis can also cause more severe disability if obstruction is precipitous. Sudden blockage can arise in vessels affected by arteriosclerosis because the physical properties of atheroma and normal tissue are dissimilar. The mismatch gives rise to shearing forces and predisposes to formation of fissures and fragments of atheroma. These fragments are liable to detach and, on entering the circulation, will block small arteries downstream. When there is incomplete detachment, the flap of material can act as a valve and cause abrupt cessation of blood flow. The likelihood of incomplete detachment is increased when there is cell death within the atheroma, as occurs when diffusion is insufficient for the metabolic needs of the atheroma.

When cholesterol is deposited within vessel walls, physical obstruction narrows the arterial vessels and increases their resistance to the flow of blood. However, resistance to flow in affected vessels is not determined exclusively by physical obstruction, since deposited cholesterol will reduce the ability of arterial muscle to relax. As has been pointed out, contraction of arterial muscle provides a physiological mechanism to regulate blood flow and thereby affect blood pressure. When there is a need to constrict arterial vessels, appropriate chemicals are released into circulating blood or tissue fluid. The extent and intensity of such muscle contraction is counterbalanced by the relaxant effect of nitric oxide that is generated continuously by cells that line the inner surface of arterial vessels. Balancing these contractile and relaxant effects provides a system for bi-directional control of tissue perfusion, in which generation of nitric oxide is pivotal. Hence, it can be anticipated that arterial vessels will constrict at sites of cholesterol deposition since high concentrations of cholesterol will both impair the formation of nitric oxide by lining cells and diminish the ability of nitric oxide to relax arterial muscle. Once initiated, this defect becomes self-perpetuating since increased blood pressure will favour additional deposition of cholesterol. It follows therefore that high plasma levels of LDL-cholesterol will be able to sustain high blood pressure.

Perception of a role for cholesterol deposits in generating and sustaining high blood pressure is attractive, for it explains an association between high blood pressure and arteriosclerosis and anticipates accumulation of platelets and white cells as a prelude to inappropriate growth of arterial muscle at sites of cholesterol deposition. Interlinking arteriosclerosis with high blood pressure in this way also explains an unexpected property of statins. Statins have been used extensively to achieve selective inhibition of an enzyme that critically controls the synthesis of cholesterol throughout the body. Hence, drugs in this category forestall the onset and retard the progression of arteriosclerosis. Although statins are not diuretic and have no direct effect on the heart, kidney or arterial muscle, they may reduce blood pressure as effectively as drugs that act on reflex systems known to control blood pressure. It seems likely therefore that the capacity of statins to promote blood pressure reduction stems from a capacity to break the cycle of self-promotion of high blood pressure that is a feature of cholesterol deposition.

2.8   High blood pressure and body mass

- Individuals who are overweight or obese are likely to develop high blood pressure
- Abdominal fat may compresses nerves that supply the kidney
- Fat cells release hormones that increase blood pressure
- Reducing body mass causes blood pressure to fall
- Individuals from isolated communities have low body mass and do not experience high blood pressure
- An urban lifestyle increases both body mass and blood pressure

Three lines of evidence link increased body weight to high blood pressure. Firstly, individuals who are obese (BMI >30 kg/m^2) or overweight (BMI 25-30 kg/m^2) are more likely to have high blood pressure and will experience strokes and coronary heart attacks more frequently than subjects who are not overweight (BMI <25 kg/m^2). Accordingly, a high proportion (65-75%) of obese or overweight adults will have a usual blood pressure that already warrants use of drugs to lower blood pressure. Secondly, overweight individuals who lose weight will experience a fall in blood pressure that is proportional to weight loss. In pooled data from 25 clinical trials when an averaged reduction of systolic (4.4 mm of mercury) and diastolic (3.6 mm of mercury) pressures parallels averaged reduction of body mass (5.1 kg). Thirdly, non-acculturated individuals, who exist on subsistence diets and are exceptionally slim (BMI <19 kg/m^2) have low blood pressures and rarely, if ever, experience strokes or coronary heart attacks. On adopting an urban lifestyle, such individuals eat excessive amounts of energy-rich foods and, as BMI rises, there is an increase of blood pressure. The prevalence of high blood pressure amongst these individuals and vulnerability to strokes or coronary heart attacks eventually merge with those of the host urban community.

It is well known that load-bearing joints in overweight individuals have an increased vulnerability to arthritis. If normal individuals carry a loaded rucksack, they can simulate this extra bodyweight and will experience sensations that make this problem intelligible. No comparable simulation will illustrate how increased body mass affects blood pressure. The closest parallel is provided by the later stages of pregnancy when, in addition to increased

BMI, there is a progressive increase of blood pressure. The "metabolic disease", which is now commonplace in developed countries, is an alternative condition in which body weight and blood pressure rise in parallel. In the metabolic disease, excess fat accumulates within the abdominal cavity to give a characteristically high ratio of waist to hip circumferences. Such individuals become insensitive to insulin and have relatively high blood levels of glucose and triglycerides as well as a reduced concentration of HDL-cholesterol. Nevertheless it is not understood why high blood pressure should be a characteristic of this syndrome. Conceivably, blood pressure might become raised if abdominal fat pads restrict the flow of blood into the kidneys and cause a compensatory secretion of renin. Should high blood pressure arise in this way, filtration units in the kidney will be lost progressively and high blood pressure will thereby be intensified. Significantly, metabolic disease is prevalent in persons whose diminished growth as a foetus resulted in a low birth weight so that their kidneys are proportionately small. With ready access to food as adults, the resulting excessive body mass is liable to overburden their small kidneys.

It is possible that processes unrelated to kidney function also contribute to the high blood pressure of subjects who are overweight or obese. Although fat cells have long been viewed as simple receptacles for storage of fat, it has been established more recently that fat cells can secrete diverse local hormones. Unsurprisingly, the total amount of fat in the body is paralleled by an increased concentration of these substances in blood. Leptin is one such local hormone whose concentrations rise with increased body mass. Secretion of leptin is a reaction to excessive eating and there is excessive secretion of leptin in mice that are genetically predisposed to obesity. Secretion of leptin might also determine raised blood pressure since intravenous injection of leptin raises the blood pressure of normal animals. It is therefore possible that formation of leptin contributes to the increase of blood pressure that is observed in the metabolic syndrome and in other forms of obesity. The ability of leptin to raise blood pressure is not a consequence of direct contraction of arterial muscle nor does leptin mimic, or influence, the renin-angiotensin system. Elevation of blood pressure by leptin is rather an indirect effect that stems from increased discharge of constrictor substances from sympathetic nerve terminals.

There can be no doubt that a high body mass increases the likelihood of high blood pressure. Even so, the physiological basis of this association is not yet adequately understood. The level of BMI that is used to predict onset of vulnerability to high blood pressure has therefore been selected arbitrarily. On the strength of surveys in large populations, it is expected that holding BMI at, or below, 22 kg/m^2 is likely to prevent, and will certainly retard, progression to high blood pressure.

2.9   High blood pressure and diet

- Excessive consumption of high energy food raises blood pressure by increasing body mass
- Increased intake of salt raises blood pressure by increasing blood volume
- Regular consumption of other salts, fish oils or garlic will reduce high blood pressure
- High blood pressure will be reduced on adopting a diet, of fruits, vegetables, low-fat diary products with very little animal fat or sugar

It has long been recognised that certain dietary habits are linked to development of high blood pressure. Most obvious is the development of high blood pressure simply because of the calorific imbalance that arises from excessive eating. When food intake is excessive, high blood pressure cannot be attributed to specific components of food, even though particular foods may increase or decrease usual blood pressure.

From amongst the other dietary constituents that might increase blood pressure, much attention has been given to dietary salt (sodium chloride). Measurement of the prevalence of high blood pressure in five distinct populations (northern Japan, southern Japan, North America, Marshall Island and Alaska) provides a comparison of dietary habits that range from near exclusion to an exceptional intake (See Figure 9). The intake of salt correlated with the incidence of high blood pressure. This association could explain the prevalence of haemorrhagic strokes in Northern Japan. It could also explain an absence of strokes amongst Yanomamo Indians, non-acculturated tribes that live at the border between Venezuela and Brazil. Their "no-salt" culture is associated with usual blood pressures of 100 (systolic) and 64 (diastolic) mm of mercury. This conclusion is straightforward but may not apply to all circumstances since Kuna Indians of Panama have a low level of blood pressure that does not rise with age, yet have a liking for salt and routinely include considerable amounts in their diet.

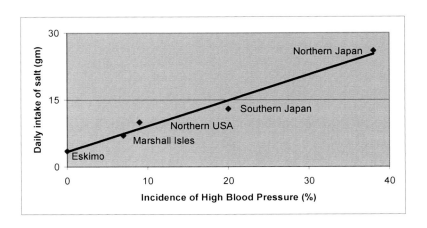

Figure 9. Correlation between salt intake and high blood pressure.

The inference that addition of salt to the diet can increase usual blood pressure has been confirmed experimentally. By eating food that was enriched with salt, chimpanzees experienced raised blood pressures over a period of 15 months. Pressures increased to 33 (systolic) and 10 (diastolic) mm of mercury and these increases were reversed by withholding supplementary salt. Corresponding studies in humans are hampered by a need to ensure that volunteers would tolerate imposition of such a diet for a long period; furthermore, such studies might be precluded by ethical considerations. Instead of investigating the effect of a fixed intake of salt, blood pressure has been measured regularly in volunteers who increased, or decreased, their intake of dietary salt. Inevitably, such studies are compromised by unrecorded dietary modifications that seek to compensate for reduced palatability. For instance, it is difficult to avoid increased consumption of fruit and vegetables over long periods when salt is being withheld and the high content of potassium and nitrate in these foods will reduce blood pressure. Despite the difficulties posed by having to conduct such studies, there is now a broad consensus that intake of sodium should be limited to 2,400 mg per day (i.e. 6 gm of salt). Adhering to this recommendation may lower usual blood pressure by 4-5 mm of mercury.

By comparison with the effect of dietary salt in animals, an averaged reduction of 4-5 mm of mercury is a modest effect. However averaged reduction is attenuated by measurements from those individuals whose blood pressure is unaffected by dietary salt. This insensitivity can be detected in >40% of patients with high blood pressure and >50% of normal individuals. Sensitivity to dietary salt may stem from reflex mechanisms that control the amount of nor-adrenaline released during vasoconstriction. These reflexes could have been invaluable when access to dietary salt was inconsistent and when compensating for a reduced intake of salt by reflex changes of blood pressure would not then have been contraindicated.

Salts of potassium and calcium are present in the diet and also influence blood pressure. Salts of potassium reduce usual blood pressure and are constituents of fruit and vegetables. Within a group of 2,500 patients, addition of supplementary potassium to the diet reduced blood pressure by 3 (systolic) and 2 (diastolic) mm of mercury. Similar considerations apply to calcium salts, which are abundant in animal bones as well as in many plant tissues. In a group of 1,200 patients with high blood pressure, addition of supplementary calcium to the diet caused systolic blood pressure to fall by almost 2 mm of mercury. Nitrates are will also lower blood pressure. These salts are constituents of plant tissues and are stored in considerable quantities by beetroot, lettuce and other cultivated vegetables. On contact with bacteria in the mouth, nitrates are converted into nitrites, which relax arterial muscle. Because of this transformation into nitrites, consumption of beetroot may lower systolic blood pressure by more than 10 mm of mercury.

Increased consumption of specific types of food can also result in reduced blood pressure. Pooled evidence from 90 studies demonstrates that consumption of fish oil (4 gm each day) reduces blood pressure by 2.1 (systolic) and 1.6 (diastolic) mm of mercury. Other dietary factors have comparable effects. For instance, 11 from 25 studies reveal that consumption of powdered garlic (600-900 mg each day) reduces blood pressure by 8.4 (systolic) and 7.3 (diastolic) mm of mercury. It can be anticipated that individual food constituents will interact synergistically, so that combinations of foods will be more effective. An example of this approach is provided by DASH (dietary control to stop hypertension). In this diet, fruits, vegetables, low-fat diary products, whole grains, poultry, fish and nuts predominate and consumption of fats, red meat sweet-tasting items is minimal. By eight weeks, blood pressure may have been reduced by 11 (systolic) and 6 (diastolic) mm of mercury. In part, this outcome may be a reflection of reduced intake of sodium (3 gm per day), increased intake of magnesium (173%), potassium (150%), fibre (240%) and protein (30%) and an increased intake of vitamins A, B, C, E, folate, riboflavin, phosphorous and zinc.

2.10   Diabetes and high blood pressure

- Diabetes arises if secretion of insulin is insufficient to control the concentration of glucose in blood
- Diabetes can also result from tissues becoming insensitive to insulin
- High concentrations of glucose promote damage to arterial vessels which makes them more vulnerable to pulses of high pressure
- Subjects who are resistant to the actions of insulin are more likely to have high blood pressure
- In diabetic patients, systolic pressures greater than 120 mm of mercury and diastolic pressures greater than 70 mm of mercury increase the likelihood of sudden death, as well as the risk of vascular complications

The human body maintains a concentration of glucose within blood and tissue fluids that is relatively constant. This regulation of glucose concentration is primarily determined by insulin, a hormone that is secreted directly into blood from specialised cells located within the pancreas. When the concentration of glucose in blood exceeds 1 mg/ml, insulin is secreted and causes the liver and skeletal muscles to abstract glucose from blood for storage. Glucose is stored by being assembled into larger molecules of glycogen. Storage is reversible and, if the concentration of glucose in blood falls below 1 mg/ml, glucose can be released from stored glycogen. Such bi-directional control avoids accumulation of glucose in plasma during digestion, yet ensures that adequate amounts of glucose can readily be made available during physical activity. A feature of this form of regulation is that it avoids exposure of tissues to excessively high, or excessively low, concentrations of glucose.

In the absence of insulin, the process of digestion causes glucose to surge into blood. Although glucose is not normally present, it will enter urine as the concentration rises in plasma. Hence, detection of glucose in urine is diagnostic diabetes and testing for glucose in urine provides a simple test for this disease. Now that measurement of glucose in blood can be easily achieved, the use of urine for indirect testing has been superseded by measurement of glucose in blood. Such measurements are straightforward and portable devices that allow automatic measurement of the concentration of glucose in blood are widely available.

Secretion of insulin is diminished if the specialised cells that generate this hormone are damaged (Type I diabetes). Once rare, this form of defective control is being detected in children and young adults with increasing frequency. Precisely how the cells that secrete insulin are damaged so selectively has yet to be established. The relatively precipitous onset that is usual in type I diabetes would be consistent with an infection or an acute immunological reaction. The alternative form (Type II diabetes) arises when liver and muscle cells lose their ability to respond to insulin and therefore fail to abstract surplus glucose from circulating blood. Such unresponsiveness does not have a sudden onset and may reflect gradual biochemical changes that accompany increased body mass. Type II diabetes has long been known to be prevalent amongst middle-aged or elderly individuals and is now being detected in young persons who eat excessively. If Type II diabetes is not being treated, eating can produce concentrations of glucose in blood that match the excessive concentrations observed during Type I diabetes. Hence, despite being determined by quite different cellular mechanisms, both forms of diabetes will produce similar symptoms. Either form of diabetes may be detected unexpectedly when concentrations of glucose are being measured routinely in samples of plasma.

High blood pressure will be detected in approximately 30% of Type I diabetics and in 50-80% of Type II diabetics. Although the onset of diabetes is not determined by changed blood pressure, diabetes and high blood pressure often co-exist. Furthermore, subtle defects of blood glucose control can often be detected when patients have high blood pressure. Such close association has prompted suggestion that resistance to insulin could be a primary determinant of high blood pressure. Unusually, it is possible to make a direct test of this hypothesis by using metformin, which increases the sensitivity of liver and muscle cells to circulating insulin. Metformin reduces the incidence of strokes and it might be presumed that such protection might stem from a reduction of blood pressure. However, metformin does not influence usual blood pressure and it must be concluded that protection from strokes stems from some other property. Effectively, this observation excludes the possibility that high blood pressure is a consequence of changed insulin sensitivity.

Defective control of the concentration of glucose in blood causes vascular damage. These structural changes are not caused by raised blood pressure but they nonetheless make vessels more vulnerable to pulses of high blood pressure. Consequently, vascular complications are a feature of diabetes and these will become more frequent and more pronounced as blood pressure rises. It is for this reason that diabetics have an increased risk of strokes and coronary artery disease and more frequent vascular disease in the kidney, eye and skin. Although established with less certainty, it is likely that the damage to sensory nerve endings in diabetes is also accelerated and intensified by periods of high blood pressure.

Since increased blood pressure intensifies vascular complications of diabetes, it is to be expected that reducing usual blood pressure should decrease the frequency and severity of vascular complications in this disease. The protective effect of lowering usual blood pressure is appreciable and a reduction of systolic blood pressure of 10 mm of mercury diminishes the overall risk of vascular complications by 12% and the risk of death by 15%. Such protection extends across all pressures in excess of 140 (systolic) and 90 (diastolic) mm of mercury and extends moreover into pressure levels that would otherwise be regarded as normal. As it is not possible to specify a threshold, it is sensible for diabetic patients to reduce their usual blood pressure as far as is practicable.

Control of high blood pressure is therefore especially important for patients with diabetes. It is usual for such patients to attempt weight loss, increased exercise and a reduced intake of sodium in addition to using drugs to lower blood pressure. Data from five large trials in diabetic patients show that between 3 and 5 drugs may have to be used to maintain pressure at, or below, 130 (systolic) and 85 (diastolic) mm of mercury. It is important for diabetic patients to ensure that nocturnal blood pressures are maintained at, or below, these levels in order to avoid damage to arteries in the eye and the kidney.

2.11 High blood pressure in pregnancy

- During normal pregnancy, blood pressure initially falls and then rises progressively until termination
- In 10% of pregnancies, there is no fall initially and blood pressure continues to rise until termination
- Only very rarely does raised blood pressure persist following termination of a pregnancy
- After high blood pressure in pregnancy, there is a slightly increased risk of high blood pressure in later life
- Excessively high blood pressure during pregnancy may lead to abnormal perfusion of the placenta and adverse effects on the foetus
- Excessively high blood pressure during pregnancy increases the risk of stroke in the mother

In normal pregnancies, it is usual for blood pressure to fall by 5 to 10 mm of mercury during the early stage. As pregnancy proceeds, this fall is nullified and pressures rise steadily until term. In a substantial minority of mothers (10%), there is no initial fall and blood pressure rises continuously from 20 weeks onward to reach levels that would merit diagnosis of high blood pressure. Such changes are likely in one of three first pregnancies. When compared with the exceedingly low incidence of high blood pressure if young women are not pregnant, the prevalence of high blood pressure during pregnancy must be recognised as extraordinary.

Development of high blood pressure during pregnancy can sometimes be anticipated because of pre-existing kidney disease (e.g. renal stenosis). There will also be a very small number of mothers already proceeding to high blood pressure, irrespective of their pregnancy. However, in the vast majority raised blood pressure will be a direct consequence of confinement. As the increase of blood pressure in pregnancy resolves fully at birth or termination, it can be assumed that it is a direct consequence of physiological changes that occur during pregnancy. As might be expected, this increase is transient and only marginally raises the risk of high blood pressure in later life, excepting amongst those who have experienced pre-eclampsia.

In a normal pregnancy, blood pressure changes are typically modest, falling initially and rising as termination approaches (See Figures 10 & 11). In mothers who progress to high blood pressure, the initial fall is not evident. Instead, blood pressure rises inexorably and progresses until pressures match those of patients with high blood pressure. In the absence of additional symptoms, such high blood pressure will be diagnosed as "gestational hypertension". Similar changes of blood pressure occur during pre-eclampsia but, in this condition, abnormalities of kidneys, liver and brain as well as of blood coagulation arise concurrently. In both gestational hypertension and in pre-eclampsia, high blood pressure resolves promptly after termination of the pregnancy. It might reasonably be concluded that the presence of a foetus and placenta determines high blood pressure both in pre-eclampsia and in gestational high blood pressure. Both conditions are readily detected as a progressive rise of blood pressure in the early stages of pregnancy and can be differentiated from a normal pregnancy, in which blood pressure does not become raised until after the 20th week.

Development of high blood pressure during pregnancy increases the risk of strokes in the mother, in like manner to the increased risk experienced by non-pregnant individuals with high blood pressure. High blood pressure during pregnancy can pose additional problems since it is liable to lead to abnormal perfusion of the placenta, thereby placing the foetus at risk. Because high blood pressure is encountered so frequently during pregnancy, blood pressure is monitored routinely by the midwife in order to guard against maternal or foetal complications. Once high blood pressure is recognised in a pregnant mother, laboratory and other investigations will be used to differentiate gestational hypertension from pre-eclampsia. Early detection of either condition is important since pressures in excess of 170 (systolic) or 110 (diastolic) mm of mercury may necessitate rapid intervention to avoid strokes and convulsions.

Attempts to account for high blood pressure during pregnancy tend to replicate explanations that have been, or are being, developed to explain high blood pressure in the general population. Suggestion that high blood pressure in pregnancy could be secondary to insulin resistance is a viewpoint that parallels attempts to link high blood pressure with glucose metabolism in the metabolic syndrome. Superficial similarities do not warrant presumption of an underlying mechanism common to both conditions and resistance to insulin does not account for either form of high blood pressure. A striking feature of high blood pressure in pregnancy is that it is almost invariably transient, whereas in the metabolic syndrome high blood pressure is likely to be persistent. Nevertheless it is possible that elimination of high blood pressure within hours of loss of the foetus and placenta might have a counterpart in the slow reduction of blood pressure that accompanies gradual weight loss in overweight individuals. Support for this viewpoint is the finding that increased concentrations of leptin parallel increased blood pressure in pregnant mothers as well as in overweight individuals. However, it has yet to be established whether formation of leptin contributes to the rise of blood pressure in pregnancy.

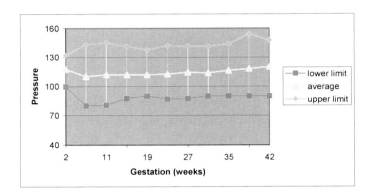

Figure 10. Averaged systolic pressure, with upper and lower bounds, for a group of circa 1000 pregnancies.

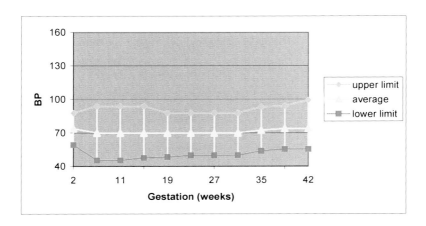

Figure 11. Averaged diastolic pressure, with upper and lower bounds, for a group of circa 1000 pregnancies.

3. Treatment of high blood pressure

3.1   What levels of blood pressure merit treatment?

- Since no usual blood pressure is representative, thresholds for diagnosis and treatment of high blood pressure are arbitrary
- Thresholds for introducing drugs to lower blood pressure are typically 140 (systolic) and 90 (diastolic) mm of mercury
- Thresholds for recommending lifestyle changes to lower blood pressure are 130 (systolic) and 85 (diastolic) mm of mercury
- Thresholds for increased risk of strokes and coronary heart attacks are 115 (systolic) and 75 (diastolic) mm of mercury
- Most middle-aged and almost all elderly adults would benefit from attempting to retard upward progression of their blood pressure

For many constituents of blood, concentrations lie consistently within narrow ranges that might reasonably be considered normal for each substance. For instance, the concentration of glucose in blood typically lies between 0.8 and 1.2 mg per ml. Because this is a narrow range, solitary measurements of blood glucose suffice to detect diabetes with considerable certainty. By way of contrast, measurements of blood pressure in individuals from developed countries do not reveal a narrow range of pressures. Consequently, solitary measurements cannot be used for diagnosis of high blood pressure in a way that is comparable with diagnosis of diabetes. In the context of diagnosis, measurements of blood pressure and measurements of many chemical constituents of blood are dissimilar.

Failure of measurements of blood pressure to reveal a narrow range of pressures that might be considered normal, has prompted a search for an alternative way to define normal blood pressure. To this end, the frequency of strokes and coronary heart attacks has been measured in tens of thousands of subjects over several years. In such surveys, blood pressure is measured at recruitment and at intervals thereafter, whilst the frequency of strokes and coronary heart attacks is monitored by reference to medical records or death certificates. Such surveys reveal that modestly increased blood pressure is associated with a substantially increased risk of strokes or coronary heart attacks. For instance, data pooled from nine studies that lasted between 6 and 25 years establish that a rise of usual diastolic blood pressure of 5 mm of mercury increases the risk of strokes by 34% and of coronary heart attacks by 21%. These extra risks are the same whether diastolic pressure has increased from 76 to 81 mm of mercury or from 100 to 105 mm of mercury.

Frequencies of strokes and coronary heart attacks are directly proportional to usual blood pressure. Hence, increased risk is predictable and such predictions are easy to verify. On the other hand, it is quite difficult to define pressure levels that are without such increased risk. This is because strokes and coronary heart attacks are relatively rare events in subjects who are classified as healthy. Consequently, exceedingly large numbers of volunteers have to be recruited to ensure that estimated rates will be reliable. Despite huge effort, it is not possible to decide whether the risk of strokes and coronary heart attacks is increased by blood pressures that are less than 115 (systolic) or 75 (diastolic) mm of mercury. Currently, these are taken as thresholds for increased risk since, above these levels, risk increases inexorably. A need to discriminate between increased risks at higher pressures and the unchanging risks at lower pressures can be aided by the "logistic spline technique". Using this technique delineates different thresholds for sub-groups, selected according to gender, age or other characteristics. For instance, the incidence of strokes is just beginning to rise when systolic pressure exceeds 140 mm of mercury for individuals aged between 44 and 54 years. For individuals aged between 55 and 64 years or between 65 and 74, the corresponding thresholds approach or even equal 160 mm of mercury (See Figures 12, 13 & 14). The existence of different thresholds for different age groups questions the practice of using a systolic pressure of 140 mm of mercury as an invariant upper limit for normal systolic pressure. Corresponding arguments hold for measurements of diastolic pressure. Defining these thresholds has a practical implication since it is usual to justify prescription of drugs that lower blood pressure as a life-long treatment to reduce or abolish such increased risk.

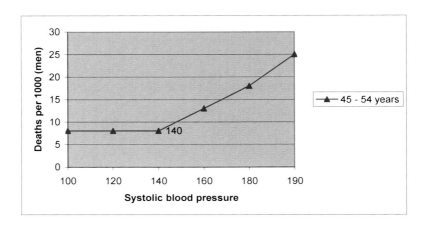

Figure 12. Threshold for increased risk of death from stroke for individuals aged between 45 and 54 defined by a logistic spline plot.

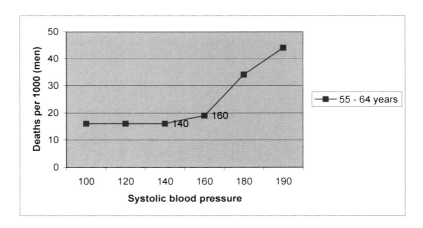

Figure 13. Threshold for increased risk of death from stroke for individuals aged between 55 and 64 defined by a logistic spline plot.

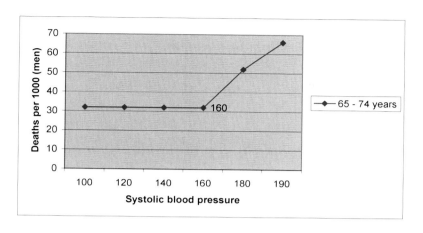

Figure 14. Threshold for increased risk of death from stroke for individuals aged between 65 and 74 defined by a logistic spline plot.

Guidelines from the British Hypertension Society advise that pressures in excess of 160 (systolic) or 100 (diastolic) mm of mercury necessitate introduction of drug therapy as treatment for high blood pressure. For pressures between 140 and 160 (systolic) and 90 and 100 (diastolic) mm of mercury, drug therapy is recommended if there is co-existing diabetes, a substantially increased risk of cardiovascular disease or of organ damage that might be linked to high blood pressure. Other authorities favour introduction of drug therapy at lower pressures. For instance, the Joint National Committee on Prevention, Evaluation and Treatment of High Blood Pressure (a coalition of leaders from 46 professional, public, voluntary and federal heath care agencies in USA) recommend introduction of drug therapy if blood pressure exceeds 140 (systolic) or 90 (diastolic) mm of mercury. Their recommendation is justified by the increased risk of strokes or coronary heart attacks at these pressures. Such untoward outcomes are exaggerated by other factors. For instance, age, gender, diabetes, a previous stroke or a previous coronary heart attack will influence the risk of future strokes and heart attacks when blood pressure is raised. The frequencies of fatal stoke in different age groups demonstrate such interaction. For individuals aged between 50 and 60, the risk of death from a stroke when systolic blood pressure is 180 mm of mercury is 16-fold greater than when systolic pressure is 120 mm of mercury. For individuals who are aged between 80 and 90, risk of a fatal stroke is already high when systolic blood pressure is 120 mm of mercury and this risk is merely doubled when systolic blood pressure has risen to 180 mm of mercury. Consequently, doctors may exercise some latitude when introducing drug therapy.

When blood pressure exceeds 140 (systolic) or 90 (diastolic) mm of mercury, modifications of lifestyle will usually cause blood pressure to fall appreciably. Hence, a need for lifestyle changes is usually emphasised when drugs are being introduced to lower blood pressure. Indeed, when raised blood pressure is close to the threshold for diagnosis, a trial of lifestyle modification may be recommended. This strategy is attractive since it could defer, and may even avoid, introduction of drugs to reduce blood pressure. However, most patients will lack the considerable resolution and self-discipline that are needed to maintain lifestyle changes over long periods and consequently will breach these thresholds. As with dieting, ambition usually overshadows achievement. Hence, it is more usual to introduce a change of lifestyle as an adjunct, rather than an alternative, to prescription of drugs that lower blood pressure.

Implicit in the proposition that particular levels of blood pressure merit treatment is a presumption that lower levels do not require treatment. Observations that have linked cardiovascular ill health to usual blood pressure provide a means of checking upon this presumption. As usual blood pressures rise towards the threshold for diagnosis of high blood pressure, there are indications of latent cardiovascular ill health. This is indicated by the names used to describe these pressure levels. Blood pressures between 130 and 140 (systolic) and between 85 and 90 (diastolic) mm of mercury have been described as "high normal" whilst pressures between 120 and 130 (systolic) and between 80 and 85 (diastolic) mm of mercury are described as "normal". As "optimal" was being used concurrently if pressures were less than 120 (systolic) and 80 (diastolic) mm of mercury, "normal" should be recognised as a misnomer. Despite having been used extensively because of its convenience, such classification is nonetheless irrational: those who are categorised as "normal" or "high normal" have an increased risk of strokes and coronary heart attacks. Even those categorised as "optimal" have a risk that is greater than individuals with pressures of 115 (systolic) or 75 (diastolic) mm of mercury.

The cumulative incidence of cardiovascular disease is higher when blood pressure lies between 130 and 140 (systolic) or 85 and 90 (diastolic) mm of mercury. From 35 to 65 years, the annual increase is 0.4% (women) and 0.8% (men) and from 65 and 90 years, the annual increase is 1.8% (women) and 2.5% (men). In effect, using the term "high normal" acknowledges this increased risk. Literal interpretation of such terminology can cause treatment to be deferred and, by allowing progression of vascular damage, will increase the risk of disability or even sudden death from a stroke or a coronary heart attack. Such a misfortune became evident during screening of a group of >20,000 individuals who were not known to have cardiovascular disease. Amongst this group, individuals were classified as having high blood pressure if measurement of diastolic blood pressure exceeded 90 mm of mercury. During screening, a disproportionate number were categorised as "high normal" with pressures of 88-89 mm of mercury. It seems likely that these individuals may have welcomed exclusion from drug treatment. Yet the rate of mortality in this group was significantly higher than in the corresponding group whose pressures of 90-91 mm of mercury had led to diagnosis of "high blood pressure" and treatment with drugs.

Once it had been established that pressures above 120 (systolic) or 80 (diastolic) mm of mercury are predictive of future disease, it became necessary to revise official recommendations. In May 2003, the Joint National Committee on Prevention, Evaluation and Treatment of High Blood Pressure in USA proposed that blood pressures should not exceed 115 (systolic) and 75 (diastolic) mm of mercury. Accordingly, a revised classification was introduced to indicate the increased risk of these lower pressures (See Table 5). The committee also recommended regular measurement of blood pressure in all individuals from the age of 21 years onwards. In the revised classification, optimal pressures are now only slightly greater than the levels that are used to define low blood pressure - when pressure does not exceed 110 (systolic) or 60 (diastolic) mm of mercury. It is to be expected that further downward revision could exclude normal blood pressure as a distinct category.

Blood pressure (mm of mercury)		Descriptor	
Systolic	Diastolic	Traditional	Revised (2003)
< 115	< 75	Not included	Optimal
< 120	< 80	Optimal	Pre-hypertensive
120-129	80-84	Normal	Pre-hypertensive
130-139	85-89	High Normal	Pre-hypertensive
> 140	> 90	High	High

Table 5. Revised classification of blood pressure categories following recognition that risk of death from stroke or coronary heart attack increases significantly when blood pressure exceeds 115 (systolic) or 75 (diastolic) mm mercury

It is difficult to establish a level of blood pressure that should be considered normal. Relating usual blood pressure to the occurrence of strokes and coronary heart attacks is one way to resolve this difficulty. This relationship justifies using systolic pressures of 160 or 140 mm of mercury as a threshold for introducing drugs that lower blood pressure. Although systolic pressures less than 140 mm of mercury do not usually trigger drug treatment, these levels cannot be considered normal since the risk of strokes or coronary heart attacks amongst such individuals is increased substantially. Because of this increased risk, all individuals with systolic pressures between 115 and 140 mm of mercury might be classified as in need of some form of treatment to lower their blood pressure. As more than half of adults in developed countries will have systolic pressures in this range, it would not be possible to offer treatment. Even developed countries with the most advanced facilities, such huge numbers would overwhelm monitoring facilities. At present, regular monitoring is therefore only available for patients whose high blood pressure coexists with cardiovascular complications. Regular monitoring is likely only when patients have detectable damage to target organs, have diabetes, or are at increased risk of cardiovascular disease. The much larger group with pre-hypertension is disregarded by the expedient of classification. Thus, whether classified as "high normal", "normal", or "optimal" or by the contemporary equivalent "pre-hypertensive", regular monitoring of their blood pressure would not be contemplated. Self-monitoring may be the only solution to their need. It is now recognised that reducing blood pressure will decrease the risk of strokes or coronary heart attacks irrespective of whether blood pressure is very high or close to normal. As the majority of adults have a usual systolic blood pressure that exceeds 120 mm of mercury, reduction of usual blood pressure could benefit most adults (See Figures 15 & 16).

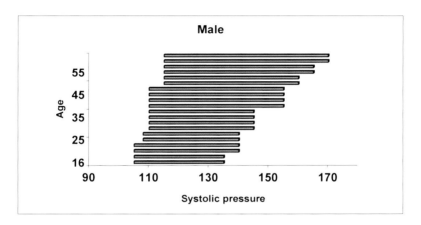

Figure 15. Range of systolic pressure for males at different ages.

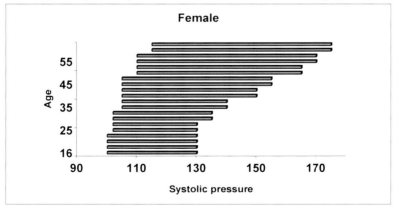

Figure 16. Range of systolic pressure for females at different ages.

A changed diet, reduced salt intake, increased aerobic exercise and weight loss will help to reduce blood pressure and might usefully be augmented by drugs that lower blood pressure. In developed countries, there is a tendency for concerns about untoward side effects to retard introduction of novel vaccines or preventive drugs in almost all area of medicine. Reservation over the regular use of drugs to prevent high blood pressure is to be expected. Those holding such opinions should be aware that serious damage to vital organs will be accumulating silently whilst blood pressure is being maintained at levels that are usual in pre-hypertension and early hypertension (See Figure 8). Hence, avoiding this form of preventive therapy is ill judged since drugs used currently used to lower blood pressure share impressive safety profiles. By way of comparison, there is little reservation over the prospective use of novel drugs to reduce body mass, even though decades would be needed before such drugs could acquire safety profiles comparable with those of drugs that are used presently to control high blood pressure.

Using drugs as a preventive therapy for strokes and coronary heart attacks would benefit many individuals who, in present circumstances, receive well meaning advice but are denied drug treatment. If such drugs were available in pharmacies without any need for prescription, this approach would not be a burden to primary care. Daily use of a "polypill" could lower blood pressure and heart rate, suppress activation of platelets, reduce plasma levels of serum homocysteine and of the low density lipoprotein carrier for cholesterol. It is predicted that adopting such a strategy could reduce the risk for strokes and coronary heart attacks amongst all individuals aged 55 or more and thereby increase averaged life expectancy by up to 11 years. Acceptance of a formulation of five established drugs is a pre-requisite of this strategy and, predictably, such proposal has induced a vigorous debate. Use of statins to prevent accumulation of cholesterol has been readily accepted and these drugs are now available without prescription. As statins can be shown to counter high blood pressure, they may provide a precedent for widespread use of drugs to prevent a progressive increase of blood pressure.

3.2 Reduction of blood pressure by lifestyle

- Intense physical activity coupled with a limited intake of food will reduce blood pressure
- Eating more fruit and vegetables reduces blood pressure by increasing the intake of potassium, nitrate and calcium
- Regular consumption of fish oil, garlic or of dairy peptides can reduce high blood pressure
- Breathing exercises that counter stress will reduce high blood pressure
- Avoiding consumption of alcohol will lower blood pressure and is also effective by reducing body weight
- Cessation of smoking has no immediate effect on usual blood pressure but, over time, is effective by avoiding arterial damage

Joints that are over-extended, overloaded or subjected to repetitive flexion and extension are likely to become damaged. The resulting swelling and tenderness induce an involuntary immobilisation. This immobilisation resolves the swelling and accelerates restoration of normal function. Immunological events produce comparable swelling and pain in the joints of patients with rheumatoid arthritis and immobilisation of such joints in a plaster cast will similarly resolve the swelling and pain. However, restoration of normal use offers no relief since symptoms recur with undiminished intensity.

Damage to arteries differs from damage to joints since there is neither swelling nor pain and since immobilisation is precluded. Nevertheless it is possible to reduce stresses within vessel walls by using drugs that lower usual blood pressure. The possibility therefore arises that such drugs might provide a route to recovery should the damage to vessel walls not be irreversible. Knowledge of the natural history of high blood pressure in pregnancy indicates such a window of opportunity for high blood pressure of pregnancy will wane within 24 hours of termination of pregnancy. Onset of high blood pressure in pregnancy is sharply defined whereas in other circumstances it will typically have an insidious onset that exposed arteries to raised pressures for many months or even for years. It cannot therefore be presumed that the brief exposure to high blood pressure during pregnancy is necessarily predictive for high blood pressure that has been overlooked.

When high blood pressure has existed without detection, it is likely that arterial vessels will already have developed some structural changes by the time of diagnosis. This is because growth and proliferation of arterial muscle is a physiological response of arteries to prolonged exposure to high pressure. On becoming enlarged, arterial muscle will cause the vessel wall to thicken, which will increase the resistance to flow by reducing the bore of the vessel. Such passively increased resistance is compounded by exaggerated constriction of enlarged muscles in the arterial wall. These passive and active changes combine to make periods of raised blood pressure protracted and intense, thereby raising the prospect of further arterial damage. Such vulnerability to further damage is reminiscent of joint damage, for which immobilisation can encourage repair. By analogy, there is a possibility that using lifestyle changes to lower blood pressure might avoid arterial damage. Prevention of an extension of damage is plausible. Whether lifestyle changes could reverse structural changes is more speculative. It is tempting to draw the analogy with physical injury to joints and to anticipate repair and recovery. However, analogy with rheumatoid arthritis may yet prove to be more appropriate.

Prevention, on the other hand, is supported by compelling evidence from preliterate communities that exist in isolation, unaffected by the wider world. In many such communities, individuals do not experience high blood pressure and thereby avoid strokes and coronary heart attacks. From this, it is reasonable to infer that vulnerability to strokes and coronary heart attacks might stem from lifestyle. This viewpoint is reinforced by detection of increased blood pressure when individuals from such communities leave to adopt an urban lifestyle. It is reasonable to conclude that youngsters from developed countries need to be alerted to the risk of high blood pressure and the advantage of opting for a lifestyle that combines high physical activity with a diet nearer to subsistence than is usual. By this means, they could reasonably expect to retard, and possibly arrest, progression to pre-hypertension. Amongst the middle-aged and elderly, it is likely that pre-hypertension will already have become established. For this reason, the effectiveness of lifestyle changes will depend upon reversibility of structural changes in arterial vessels. Reversibility is not excluded since regular use of statins protects from stokes and coronary heart attacks and higher doses are increasingly effective. On balance, it may be expected that lifestyle changes would slow the progression from pre-hypertension to high blood pressure. However, it must be acknowledged that evidence favouring such protection is not as convincing as the evidence of increased risk to vital organs when blood pressure is increased.

Factor	Recommendation	Reduction of systolic/ diastolic pressures (mm mercury)
Body mass	Reduce BMI to < 25	1.5/1 per kg of lost body weight
Physical activity	Aerobic exercise for > 30 minutes daily	13/8 over several weeks
Diet	Adopt a DASH diet	11/6 over several weeks
Fish oil	> 4 gm daily	2/2 over several weeks
Garlic powder	600-900 mg daily	8.5/7 over several weeks
Dairy peptides	Daily intake	7/4 over several weeks
Salt intake	< 6 gm daily	5/2 over several months
Potassium intake	Eat fresh fruit & vegetables	3/2 over several months
Nitrate intake	Eat beetroot, lettuce & other vegetables	>10 (systolic) over several weeks
Stress/anxiety	Slow, deep breathing for 15 min daily	14/8 over several weeks
Alcohol intake	<14 units/week (women) <21 units/week (men)	13 (systolic) acutely if alcohol-dependent
Smoking	Cessation	Slight increase

Table 6. Lifestyle changes that influence usual blood pressure

An absence of high blood pressure in non-acculturated communities accords with recommendation of lifestyle changes to prevent the onset and progression of high blood pressure (See Table 6). Amongst these recommendations, a changed diet might be expected to be protective since it has long been known that excess body weight is associated with an increased blood pressure. Individuals who are overweight typically have enlarged fat deposits within their abdominal cavity, which manifest as middle-aged spread. Excessive amounts of abdominal fat may physically stimulate sympathetic nerves that enter the kidney and fat cells at this site could release excessive amounts of angiotensin II. By causing retention of sodium, these processes transfer of water into plasma and oblige blood pressure to rise. It is possible that this sequence of events could be reversed by removal of excess fat from the abdominal cavity. Whether removed by surgery or by dietary changes, there will be a fall of blood pressure of 1.6 (systolic) and 1.1 (diastolic) mm of mercury for each kilogram of weight lost. Regular exercise augments this fall by up to 13 (systolic) and 8 (diastolic) mm of mercury, independently of weight loss. In many subjects with high blood pressure, dieting in combination with regular aerobic exercise is therefore a cornerstone of treatment plans.

Since dietary changes can reduce blood pressure independently of calorific intake, introduction of specific chemicals or changing the proportions of dietary constituents are alternatives to reducing total consumption of food. For instance, varying the proportion of dietary constituents may reduce high blood pressure, as when adopting a diet in which intake of fruit, vegetables and low-fat dairy products is increased and intake of saturated fats is lowered (DASH diet). Adherence to a DASH diet over an eight-week period causes blood pressure to fall by 11 (systolic) and 5.5 (diastolic) mm of mercury. Alternatively, consumption of specific foods can be used to achieve significant reduction of high blood pressure, with fish oil and garlic providing well studied examples. When consuming 4 gm of fish oil regularly blood pressure may fall by 2 (systolic) and 1.5 (diastolic) mm of mercury. Daily consumption of 600-900 mg of powdered garlic has a more substantial effect, with high blood pressure being reduced by 8.5 (systolic) and 7 (diastolic) mm of mercury. Possibly, is effective by virtue of pharmacological as well as nutritional effects since powdered garlic is similarly effective whether or not blood pressure is raised. Such strongly flavoured materials as fish oil and garlic are conveniently consumed within capsules, granules or syrup. Possibly, dairy peptides may also be effective. Isoleucineproline-proline and valine-proline-proline are formed when milk protein (casein) is broken down into small fragments. Daily consumption of drinks that contain such peptides may reduce blood pressures by 7 (systolic) and 4 (diastolic) mm of mercury.

As well as reducing the total intake of food and changing the proportions of nutrients, reducing dietary salt will lower blood pressure in most individuals. Reducing the intake of salt lowers blood pressure because it allows a greater proportion of body water to be eliminated as urine. Although salt is an essential nutrient, it is often present in foods in excessive amounts, being added either to act as a preservative or to increase palatability. The current popularity of processed foods in the UK leads to a high intake of salt and it is quite usual to have a daily intake that is 50-100% greater than needed for healthy living. Reduction of salt intake is therefore an appropriate objective for individuals with high blood pressure. Restricting salt intake has a direct effect upon blood volume. In addition, avoidance of foods with a high salt content will have indirect benefits. Foods with a high salt content (e.g. crisps, pizzas etc.) are energy rich and are often consumed together with soft drinks or beers that are also energy rich. Recently, UK regulatory bodies have required that the sodium (i.e. salt) content of foods be specified on packaging to motivate avoidance. Limiting total intake of salt to 6 gm per day will lower blood pressure by 3.7-4.8 (systolic) and 0.9-2.5 (diastolic) mm of mercury. These averaged reductions are not necessarily representative, since blood pressure is very sensitive to salt intake in some individuals but blood pressure remains unchanged in others.

Increasing the intake of potassium can compensate for a loss of palatability when sodium is withheld. Such supplementary potassium will reduce usual blood pressure but may have an adverse interaction with their prescribed drugs. Potassium supplements could also pose problems if kidney function is impaired. Hence, increased intake of potassium is best achieved by including a higher proportion of fruit and vegetables in the diet. Such a change of diet will also increase the intake of nitrate and calcium which lower blood pressure without adverse effects on the kidneys and without interaction with the drugs that control high blood pressure.

Alcohol is another food source that can affect blood pressure. Alcoholic beverages are derived from sugar and have a high calorific content. Hence, avoidance of alcoholic drinks will contribute to overall weight loss and thereby will reduce blood pressure indirectly. However, in addition to serving as a source of energy, alcohol has pharmacological effects that can influence usual blood pressure. Ingestion of modest amounts of alcohol will reduce blood pressure by relaxing the muscular wall of arterial vessels. This direct effect is augmented by effects on the brain that manifest as contentment. Effects upon the brain will counter stress and decrease the discharge of local hormones from sympathetic nerves. Set against these effects of modest quantities of alcohol is a prevalence of high blood pressure amongst those who consume excessive amounts of alcohol. When alcohol is consumed to excess, blood pressure rises by an amount that parallels the amount of alcohol circulating in blood. The capacity of alcohol to produce increased blood pressure can be revealed in individuals who regularly drink to excess, by measuring blood pressure at regular intervals during a 24-hour period of abstinence. When alcohol is withheld, 3 out of 4 will experience a fall in systolic blood pressure that exceeds 10 mm of mercury. However, as for salt, excessive consumption will increase blood pressure of some individuals but leave others unaffected. For those with high blood pressure, the effect of modest consumption of alcoholic beverages is not distinguishable from abstinence. Even so, excessive consumption should be avoided, since it is associated with an increased risk of strokes and coronary heart attacks.

Smoking of tobacco often parallels consumption of alcohol. However, whereas the effects of alcohol are predominantly nutritional, effects of tobacco are exclusively pharmacological and toxicological. Tobacco smoke rapidly introduces nicotine into the blood that fills the heart. On delivery to small arteries, nicotine can contract muscle in the vessel wall. For instance, entry of nicotine into arterial blood causes a precipitous fall of temperature in forearm skin as a result of constriction of small arteries that supply capillary vessels near to the surface of skin. Constriction may stem from a direct effect of nicotine on muscles in the wall of these arteries or may be an indirect effect due to arrival of nerve impulses from the brain. Whether direct or indirect, this effect of nicotine on arterial constriction is transient. Hence, although cessation of smoking is followed by a slight increase of usual blood pressure, smoking of tobacco has no appreciable effect in the short term. Over time, smoking does impact on high blood pressure by accelerating arteriosclerosis. This condition increases vulnerability to high blood pressure and the risk of strokes and coronary heart attacks is tripled if patients have moderately raised blood pressure. High usual blood pressure should alert individuals who smoke to an imminent risk of severe illness or even sudden death. This awareness may motivate them to desist from smoking.

Stressful situations induce a release of adrenaline and nor-adrenaline from the adrenal glands and can both accelerate and prolong the discharge of nor-adrenaline from sympathetic nerves. Blood pressure can be expected to rise in part because of constriction of arterial muscle and in part because of a loss of sensitivity of reflexes that are used to counter increased blood pressure. Predictably, stressful situations will occur more frequently whilst at work than during days at rest. Nevertheless, stressful situations are not peculiar to the workplace and may arise during travel or even during domestic activities. For those who work in an office, a burst of violent physical activity will considerably exceed even the highest levels of stress that arise in the workplace. For instance, removal of large quantities if snow from a driveway during cold weather is intensely stressful and, for sedentary workers, is infrequently associated with coronary heart attacks. If stress is suspected as a source of high blood pressure, active efforts can be made to reduce its effects. For instance, periods of slow breathing (<10 breaths per minute) with prolonged exhalation can be used. Breathing in this way for a period of 15-minutes each day for 8 weeks may reduce blood pressure by up to 14 (systolic) and 8 (diastolic) mm of mercury.

3.3   Reduction of blood pressure by drugs

- Drugs that are used to combat high blood pressure comprise six categories
- Each category interacts with a distinct physiological mechanism
- Changes of rate and force of heart muscle contraction, constriction of arterial vessels and total blood volume can separately lower usual blood pressure

Blood is comprised of a mixture of cells and fluid, contained within a closed network of tubing. Arterial vessels are used to conduct blood under pressure into very fine capillary vessels whose walls are sufficiently permeable to allow exchange of gases, transfer of nutrients and elimination of waste from tissues. Because materials are transferred across a capillary wall by diffusion, diameters of capillaries lie in the range of 10-20 microns so that exchange can be completed rapidly. To perfuse these fine vessels rapidly and uniformly, a high pressure is needed. This pressure is provided by synchronous contractions of heart muscle and is maintained by the muscular walls in the arterial network. A number of reflex mechanisms are used to maintain this pressure automatically, sometimes by diverting flow from particular organs or tissues.

Blood volume changes usually require days or weeks. Hence, the volume of blood within the arterial network is effectively held constant during day-to-day activity. Because blood volume cannot be changed abruptly, pressure changes are used to control tissue perfusion. To this end, alteration of the heart rate provides a simple way to raise or lower arterial pressure. The heartbeat is slowed by activation of parasympathetic nerve fibres that end within heart tissue. Acetylcholine from the endings of these nerves and strongly inhibits contraction of heart muscle. Once released from nerve endings, acetylcholine is destroyed within seconds by an enzyme in plasma. Hence, the effects of acetylcholine on blood pressure arise solely from actions on the heart and do not involve arterial muscle. Adrenaline and nor-adrenaline counterbalance this action of acetylcholine. Adrenaline is released into circulating blood during activation of cells within adrenal glands and from sympathetic nerve endings that lie close to the arterial wall. Consequently, adrenaline has to be present in tissue fluid or plasma for several seconds before it can change the heart beat frequency. Nor-adrenaline is released coincidentally from the endings of sympathetic nerves and constricts small arteries after traversing the tissue fluid that separates nerve endings from arterial muscle. The intense vasoconstriction produced by nor-adrenaline invokes a reflex inhibition of the heart rate by stimulating pressure receptors. Adrenaline therefore cause palpitation by accelerating the heart rate whilst nor-adrenaline produces a slight slowing of heart rate. Adrenaline and nor-adrenaline are not inactivated by blood; rather, they are eliminated by selective uptake into cells that have been adapted to remove these materials. This elimination mechanism is as selective as enzymatic destruction but operates more slowly. Hence, the duration of increased blood pressure that follows release of adrenaline and nor-adrenaline considerably exceeds the duration of reduced blood pressure that follows release of acetylcholine.

Unlike the relatively rapid changes of blood pressure that result from a changed frequency of heartbeat or from constriction of small arteries, changes of blood pressure caused by kidneys have a slower onset and are relatively protracted. Such changes are necessarily slow since they result from a gradual change of blood volume. The kidney plays a major role in controlling blood volume by sensing the inflow of blood into the kidney and secreting renin whenever inflow is reduced. On contact with blood, this enzyme initiates release of angiotensin, a peptide that stimulates release of aldosterone in order to control the amount of sodium within plasma. Retained sodium abstracts water from tissues throughout the body and hence automatically expands blood volume. Inevitably therefore, secretion of renin will increase the total volume of blood and this in turn will increase blood pressure thereby restoring kidney perfusion. Having such a chain of control helps to prevent overcompensation when inflow of blood into the kidney is reduced. For instance, transformation of angiotensin into a more potent form can be attenuated during passage through the lung. Similarly, factors other than aldosterone can be brought into play for control of sodium excretion. Thus, activation of sympathetic nerves can reduce extraction of sodium by kidney tubules; peptides released from the heart as a reaction to changed blood volume will eliminate sodium from blood; cells at the base of the brain will detect changed osmolarity (i.e. water content) of blood and will inhibit formation of urine by releasing vasopressin. Because of these interventions, several days may elapse before blood volume achieves a new equilibrium.

Small arteries are conduits that distribute blood into the fine capillaries that supply oxygen and nutrients to tissues. The resistance to flow in these vessels arises from fixed and variable components. Fixed resistance is determined by the absolute dimensions of these vessels and by the physical interaction that exists between layers of flowing blood and the inner lining of the vessel. Variable resistance arises when small arteries constrict or dilate. When nor-adrenaline is released into blood from adrenal glands and from sympathetic nerves, there is generalised constriction of arterial muscle. This arterial tone can be fine-tuned by localised release of endothelin which will cause arterial muscle to contract and by changing the rate of formation of nitric oxide at the inner surface of arteries which will cause arterial muscle to relax.

The network of controls that has been defined make it possible to understand how defective control could lead to a persisting increased blood pressure. The various constituents of this control network indicate different approaches that might be used for selecting compounds that lower blood pressure. Six distinct categories of drugs are accepted as suitable for reducing high blood pressure and, as is conventional, a prominent property is used to provide generic names for these drugs. Control of blood pressure may depend upon inhibition of angiotensin converting enzyme (ACE inhibitors), antagonism of angiotensin receptors (angiotensin receptor antagonists), antagonism of beta-adrenoceptors (beta blockers), blockade of calcium channels (calcium channel antagonists), diuresis (diuretics) or antagonism of alpha-adrenoceptors (alpha blockers).

3.4   Drugs used to reduce high blood pressure

- Inhibitors of the enzyme that converts angiotensin I to angiotensin II, diminish secretion of aldosterone
- By interacting with receptors for angiotensin II, angiotensin antagonists diminish the secretion of aldosterone
- By interacting with beta-adrenoceptors, beta blockers preclude activation of cells by adrenaline or nor-adrenaline
- Calcium channel blockers prevent calcium ions from passing into channels that permeate the outer membrane of cells
- Diuretics eliminate water by increasing the rate of formation of urine
- By interacting with alpha-adrenoceptors, alpha blockers preclude activation of cells by adrenaline or nor-adrenaline
- Statins reduce cholesterol levels in blood and reduce usual blood pressure by preventing, or reversing, arterial damage

ACE inhibitors

It has long been known that high blood pressure will develop if the inflow of blood into the renal artery of a laboratory mammal is limited surgically. Hence, it was not unexpected to find within kidney tissue a substance that increased blood pressure when injected intravenously into normal animals. Unusually, the substance responsible for increasing blood pressure in this way is an enzyme. It was given the name renin to indicate origin within the kidney. Finding an enzyme with this property was unexpected. This posed a problem for it was not immediately obvious why blood pressure should rise when an enzyme contacts blood.

Fortunately, there was a precedent. It had long been known that saliva or pancreatic secretions produce a pronounced fall of blood pressure on intravenous injection and the mechanism of this peculiar effect had already been elucidated. These glandular enzymes reduce arterial pressure by interacting with a specific protein in plasma to release a small peptide that potently relaxes arterial muscle. When this mechanism was first discovered in Germany, the peptide was named kallidin and some of the releasing enzymes were referred to as kallikreins.

Having no obvious function, this process attracted little attention. Twenty years later, this type of process was rediscovered and the peptide renamed as bradykinin, in order to indicate a slower relaxation of arterial muscle than the abrupt reaction to contemporary vasodilators, such as histamine and acetylcholine.

In small arteries, bradykinin strongly opposes constrictor tone and thereby reduces resistance to blood flow. Such a property explains why certain glandular enzymes (i.e. trypsin and salivary kallikrein) reduce blood pressure when injected intravenously into humans or animals. It was therefore anticipated that, by analogy, renin should increase blood pressure by releasing a peptide to contract arterial muscle. In accordance with this expectation, addition of renin to blood was shown to release a small peptide that strongly contracts arterial muscle and that produces sustained vasoconstriction on intravenous injection. Identified contemporaneously by two independent groups, the same peptide was referred to separately as angiotonin and hypertensin. These terms were eventually melded into angiotensin.

Angiotensin and bradykinin have opposing actions (constriction and dilatation of small arteries). Angiotensin is present in circulating blood because renin is continuously secreted into blood by the kidneys. Formation of bradykinin is intermittent, since the glandular enzymes that release bradykinin are normally isolated from circulating blood. Glandular enzymes only form bradykinin when there has been damage to salivary, pancreatic or prostate glands, as following an autoimmune reaction, infection or invasion of the gland by tumour cells. Sustained release of bradykinin is possible however there is a kallikrein in plasma that is closely related to glandular kallikeins. Plasma kallikrein will release bradykinin into plasma when activated by contact with injured tissue, including the mild injury that results from turbulent blood flow. Inevitably, there has been speculation that vasodilator effects of bradykinin might counterbalance the constrictor effects of angiotensin. However, such counterbalance could only operate close to the site of formation since bradykinin is destroyed by the lung. Thus, whereas angiotensin I is transformed into a more potent vasoconstrictor peptide on passage through the lung, bradykinin is transformed into peptide fragments that have no biological effects. Angiotensin converting enzyme within the lung therefore serves to accentuate increased blood pressure resulting from released angiotensin whilst, at the same time, protecting the body from any overall lowering of blood pressure during injury due to release of bradykinin.

By linking renin with angiotensin, it became possible to understand how reduced perfusion of the kidney could cause widespread constriction of small arteries. When first discovered, angiotensin was demonstrably the most potent constrictor of arterial vessels yet to have been identified. Not surprisingly therefore, it was widely expected that excessive formation of angiotensin would account for the high blood pressure of essential hypertension (high blood pressure of unknown origin). Despite the elegance of this concept, the amount of angiotensin in the blood of patients with high blood pressure is insufficient to contract arterial muscle. This unexpected outcome was disconcerting. It only became intelligible after it had been demonstrated that the small amounts of angiotensin present in blood are sufficient to stimulate secretion of aldosterone. This finding implies that angiotensin II could be producing high blood pressure indirectly, by increasing the volume of blood rather than by direct contraction of arterial muscle. Aldosterone retains sodium and, by compelling translocation of water from tissues into plasma, will increase blood volume and thereby raise blood pressure. Effectively therefore, the primary role of ACE within the lungs is to amplify the effect of released renin since conversion of angiotensin I into angiotensin II provides a much stronger stimulus for aldosterone release.

A pivotal role of angiotensin converting enzyme in blood pressure regulation implies that selective inhibition of this enzyme should reduce blood pressure by impairing the formation of angiotensin II. Captopril was the drug that first revealed effectiveness of ACE inhibitors in controlling high blood pressure and was superseded by enalapril, which could be used once daily. Lisinopril, ramipril, cilazapril, fosinopril, imidapril, moexipril, perinopril, quinapril and trandolapril are alternatives.

Angiotensin II antagonists

By reducing the formation of angiotensin II in the lung, ACE inhibitors can provide effective control of blood pressure. Blocking the activation of cells by angiotensin II is an alternative strategy. Although conversion occurs primarily in the lung, angiotensin I can be converted into angiotensin II at sites elsewhere in the body. Hence, it was considered possible that high blood pressure might be reduced more effectively by angiotensin II receptor antagonists than by ACE inhibitors. There is the added possibility that conservation of angiotensin II might reduce damage to the heart during high blood pressure by its physiological effects as a local hormone. The relative merits of ACE inhibitors and angiotensin II antagonists in blood pressure control could not be anticipated. However, there was confident expectation that side effect profiles of these different drug categories would not be shared. For instance, it was well established that a persisting cough could restrict the use of some ACE inhibitors and selective elimination of this side effect was an attractive goal.

The presumption that blocking the actions of angiotensin II could match inhibition of its formation for high blood pressure control has been justified. Pooled data from carefully controlled trials confirm that recommended doses of angiotensin II antagonists are slightly more effective, and have less adverse effects, than recommended doses of ACE inhibitors. It is unlikely that these differences are determined by changes in the metabolic fate of bradykinin. Although strongly vasodilator at the site of formation, this action of bradykinin is rapidly lost on dilution into venous blood. Hence, the ability of ACE inhibitors to suppress destruction of bradykinin within the lung may be inconsequential. In the special circumstance of asthma, these quite small amounts of bradykinin may suffice for airway obstruction, yet ACE inhibitors very rarely exacerbate asthma. In a substantial proportion of patients, ACE inhibitors produce cough. However, this cannot be attributed to bradykinin, since cough does not arise in asthmatics when bradykinin is used to induce airway obstruction. More probably, the propensity of certain ACE inhibitors to cause cough reflects aspects of chemical structure that are unrelated to ACE inhibition.

Losartan, candesartan, irbesartan, eprosartan, olmesartan, valsartan and telmisartan are already established as being effective in controlling blood pressure. Irbesartan may be used when there is renal failure or moderate liver failure. Olmsartan is significantly more effective in reducing diastolic pressure of patients with high blood pressure. Exceptionally, losartan promotes excretion of uric acid by the kidney and is likely to be preferred by those afflicted with gout.

Beta blockers

Discharge of adrenaline and nor-adrenaline from storage sites in the adrenal gland and localised release from nerves within the walls of small arteries will increase blood pressure. In part, this is because adrenaline and nor-adrenaline activate specific receptors (alpha-receptors & beta-receptors). Activation of either type of receptor can contract muscle in the arterial wall and both effects contribute to raised blood pressure. When beta-receptors are activated by adrenaline, the heart will contract more frequently and more intensely. This activity of heart muscle will increase the need for oxygen, which poses a problem when the heart is injured and/or when coronary blood flow is compromised. Hence, drugs that block activation of cardiac muscle by binding to beta-receptors will slow the heartbeat as a way of reducing the need for oxygen. Concurrently, these drugs block the vasodilator response that occurs when beta-receptors on arterial muscle are activated by adrenaline and nor-adrenaline. For this reason, it was predicted that the fall in blood pressure due to the slowing of the heart would be offset by diminished relaxation of arterial muscle. Hence, beta blockers were not expected to be useful for blood pressure control.

Such theoretical conjecture was eclipsed when clinical investigations revealed a significant fall of blood pressure during treatment of heart disease by beta blockers. This unexpected finding prompted reconsideration of the place of beta blockers in the treatment of high blood pressure. It quickly became apparent that these drugs are able to achieve blood pressure control, but no obvious mechanism explained effectiveness. Subsequently, it has become apparent that beta blockers diminish the frequency and intensity of sympathetic nerve discharges and hence lower usual blood pressure by reducing vasoconstriction. Beta blockers also reduce the sensitivity of pressure detectors in large arteries, thereby blunting the reflex reaction to lowered blood pressure. Additionally, an ability of beta blockers to reduce release of renin will limit the expansion of blood volume. Contributions from these indirect mechanisms could explain the net reduction of blood pressure that occurs during use of beta blockers.

The first beta blocker to be used widely in patients with high blood pressure was propranolol. This is an unselective drug that has a range of effects that do not contribute to blood pressure control, including actions in the brain. Some of these untoward consequences are avoided when beta blockers do not enter the brain and only block sub-populations of beta receptors. Despite such refinements, selective beta blockers have not provided superior control of blood pressure as compared with non-selective drugs. In most instances, neither effectiveness in blood pressure control nor the pattern and intensity of adverse effects are changed markedly by using drugs that provide a very selective blockade of beta receptors. Clearly, the precise role of beta blockade will require clarification if the untoward consequences of beta blockade are to be minimised. When beta blockade is used for treatment of high blood pressure, atenolol is likely to be preferred since it can be given once daily and has poor penetration into brain tissue. It is possible that atenolol will eventually be superseded by labetalol, carvedilol and nebivolol since these are vasodilator drugs that relax arterial muscle as well as producing beta blockade. Acebutolol, bisoprolol, celiprolol, metoprolol, nadolol, oxprenolol, pindolol and timolol are alternative betablockers.

Calcium channel blockers

A variety of cells that participate in blood pressure control are activated by calcium ions that enter special channels in the cell membrane. Within the cell, these ions are able to initiate or regulate chemical reactions. For this reason, calcium ions affect the frequency and intensity of contraction of heart muscle, the extent and duration of contraction of arterial muscle, secretion of renin from cells in the kidney and secretion of nor-adrenaline from the endings of nerve fibres. It can be inferred that blocking these channels should be able to lower blood pressure by opposing one or more of the reflexes that serve to increase usual blood pressure. Against this, blockade of calcium channels might reasonably be expected to produce effects in other cell types, many of which could be undesirable during treatment of high blood pressure. Fortunately, the characteristics of calcium channels vary from tissue to tissue and these differences have allowed selection of compounds that are predominantly effective by acting on channels that influence blood pressure control. Hence, although side effects may occur, they are no more prominent than in other drug categories used to control blood pressure.

Dihydropyridines (e.g. nifedipine, nicardipine, amlodipine) affect blood pressure by causing relaxation of arterial muscle and the duration of action of some drugs in this category (e.g. isradipine, lacidipine and lercanidipine) is sufficient to provide useful control of high blood pressure. Feldopine and nisoldipine are alternatives. Diltiazem and verapamil are drugs that block calcium channels in heart muscle and lower blood pressure by reducing output of blood from the heart. However, these drugs are preferred for treatment of angina and arrhythmia rather than for high blood pressure.

Diuretics

Since blood is contained within a closed network of tubes, any increase of blood volume will produce a corresponding increase of blood pressure. Because of this relationship, reduction of blood volume provides a straightforward way of lowering blood pressure and diuretics are a convenient way to achieve this objective. For control of high blood pressure, it is usual to favour a thiazide (e.g. bendroflumethiazide, hydrochlorthiazide) or a thiazide-like diuretic (e.g. chlortalidone, indapamide). Drugs of this type prevent sodium and chloride from being retained in kidney tubules during formation of urine. By eliminating sodium from the body they produce a proportionate reduction of blood volume. This causes blood pressure to fall as the output of blood from the heart is decreased. When use of diuretics is sustained, output of blood from the heart is slowly restored to pre-treatment levels without any loss of blood pressure control. It seems likely that this adaptation reflects a slowly developing loss of sensitivity of arterial muscle to the constrictor effect of nor-adrenaline. When responding to diuretics, increased excretion of sodium may produce side effects by eliminating potassium, calcium and magnesium. Diuretics may also cause retention of uric acid or glucose in blood and, in a minority of patients, these latter effects produce significant symptoms.

Alpha blockers

Adrenaline and nor-adrenaline are released into circulating blood following activation of endocrine cells in the adrenal gland and following stimulation of sympathetic nerve endings which lie within arterial vessel walls. They initiate contraction of arterial muscle and constrict small arteries following interaction with alpha-receptors. Blood pressure will rise and, as a corollary, blockade of these receptors will cause blood pressure to fall. Because these receptors are widely distributed throughout the body, alpha blockers are an effective treatment for high blood pressure. Although reduction of blood pressure is very effective, it has to be balanced against unwanted side-effects that can be pronounced. For instance, blockade of alpha-receptors throughout the body will impair reflexes that maintain regional blood pressure. Hence, alpha blockers are likely to cause patients to feel faint whilst standing (postural hypotension). Because of pronounced side-effects, alpha blockers are favoured when such properties can be turned to advantage. For instance, as well as relaxing arterial muscle, blockade of alpha-receptors will also relax muscles that restrict release of urine from the bladder. In males, this may be helpful if urine flow is being impaired by prostate hypertrophy. On the other hand, in women who are experiencing stress incontinence, such an effect would be unwelcome.

Doxazosin, prazosin and terazosin are selective alpha blockers that can be used once daily for control of high blood pressure.

Statins

Deposits of cholesterol distort arterial walls and the resulting folds or bulges disrupt flow of blood across the inner surface lining and increase the resistance to flow. This reduction of flow will compounded wherever there is turbulence in flowing blood. In addition to such physical effects, deposits of cholesterol will impair biochemical processes that are used to regulate flow. In small arteries, localised resistance reflects a balance between contractile and relaxant effects of local hormones. The relaxant element in this system is nitric oxide, which is generated continuously by cells that line the inner surface of arteries. Deposition of cholesterol reduces synthesis of nitric oxide and impairs its effectiveness in relaxing arterial muscle. Once initiated, this defect becomes self-perpetuating since any increase of blood pressure will favour additional deposition of cholesterol and further reduce the formation and effectiveness of nitric oxide. Predictably, such self-promotion will be exaggerated if large amounts of LDL-cholesterol are present in circulating blood. Association between high blood pressure and arteriosclerosis can be anticipated, since impaired formation of nitric oxide favours accumulation of platelets and white cells at sites of cholesterol deposition as a prelude to proliferation of arterial muscle.

Interlinking arteriosclerosis with high blood pressure in this way anticipates that statins could contribute to blood pressure control. Statins were developed as selective inhibitors of an enzyme that controls synthesis of cholesterol. It was expected that these drugs would arrest the onset and retard the progression of arteriosclerosis. It was not anticipated that statins could contribute to the control of high blood pressure since they have no direct effect on the heart, kidney or arterial muscle and are not diuretic. Yet, even when using doses selected by reference to synthesis of cholesterol, their capacity to reduce blood pressure is not far removed from that of drugs devised specifically for blood pressure control. When beta blockers were found unexpectedly to lower blood pressure effectively, they were developed as a component of blood pressure control, even though their mode of action was little understood. It may be prudent therefore to attempt a similar transformation for statins, especially as efficacy in blood pressure reduction will not be compromised by unexpected side effects.

Patients who are controlling high blood pressure by drugs that lower high blood pressure (e.g. ACE inhibitors, calcium channel blockers) have a lesser incidence of strokes and coronary heart attacks. If, in addition to using drugs for blood pressure reduction, they are also using statins, it is likely that effectiveness will not be restricted to reduced deposition of cholesterol will extend into overall blood pressure control. Because statins are widely used as a preventive therapy for arteriosclerosis, many individuals who are pre-hypertensive will be using these drugs and may be inadvertently retarding onset of high blood pressure.

Lovastatin, pravastatin, simvastatin, fluvastatin, atorvastatin and rosuvastatin are examples of statins that are used to control blood levels of cholesterol.

Drugs in combination

By using large groups of patients, it has been possible to establish doses of the different drug categories that cause equivalent reduction of blood pressure. On average, recommended doses of diuretics, beta blockers, ACE inhibitors, angiotensin II antagonists and calcium channel blockers reduce blood pressure by

9.1 (systolic) and 4.4 (diastolic) mm of mercury. These reductions are comparable with those than can be achieved by lifestyle changes. Considered in isolation, such effects might seem insufficient. However, these doses may be sufficient for use in combination. As each of these drug categories relies upon a separate mechanism of action, it is usual to prescribe these drugs in combinations that are likely to produce additive effects and may be synergistic. For instance, the elimination of excessive blood volume by diuretics will intensify the actions of beta blockers and ACE inhibitors.

Use of drugs in combination is usual and for particular categories of patients, specific combinations may be recommended. For instance, it is presumed that there will be excessive activation of the renin/angiotensin system in younger patients with high blood pressure. High blood pressure in such individuals may therefore be particularly susceptible to blockade of angiotensin formation or actions (A) or to blockade of sympathetic nerve effects by a beta blocker (B). As a corollary, it is considered more appropriate for patients with less pronounced activation of the renin/angiotensin system to use calcium channel antagonists (C) together with diuretics (D). This type of reasoning justifies certain combinations (e.g. A&C, A&D, B&C, B&D). Nevertheless, such recommendations will be disregarded if adverse effects have an overriding influence (See Table 7). For instance, use of diuretics may be avoided should patients be predisposed to gout and use of beta blockers will be avoided when the patient has respiratory symptoms. Introduction of an additional drug may be a prudent strategy during treatment of high blood pressure since use of three drugs in combination halves the risk of stroke or coronary heart attack (See Table 8).

Drug category	Adverse effects	Contraindications
ACE inhibitors	Cough Localised fluid retention Increased blood potassium Loss of taste	Pregnancy Narrowed renal arteries High blood potassium
Angiotensin receptor antagonists	Localised fluid retention Increased blood potassium	Pregnancy Narrowed renal arteries High blood potassium
Beta blockers	Bronchospasm Reduced pulse rate Cardiac failure Cold hands and feet Fatigue Erectile dysfunction Impaired control of glucose & triglycerides	Asthma Chronic obstructive pulmonary disease Heart block
Calcium channel antagonists	Swelling of lower limbs Headache Flushing Constipation	Heart block
Diuretics	Uric acid retention Urination at night	Gout
Alpha blockers	Fainting	Postural hypotension
Statins	Skeletal muscle damage	

Table 7. Adverse effects of drugs used to control high blood pressure

Consequence of high blood pressure	Reduced risk (percentages with 95% confidence estimates)		
	One drug	Two drugs	Three drugs
Stroke	29 (26-31)	49 (42-55)	63 (55-70)
Coronary heart disease	19 (17-21)	34 (29-40)	46 (39-53)

Table 8. Use of drugs, separately or in low-dose combination, to reduce the incidence of strokes and coronary heart attacks.

Timing of drug administration

Many physiological processes in the body have a 24-hour periodicity. Given the considerable differences between slumber and wakefulness, this should not be surprising. Thus, on rising in the morning, processes that have been diminished or shut down during slumber have to be reactivated. For instance, blood flow will have to increase to supply muscles used for standing and walking. This contributes to a rise of blood pressure described as the "morning surge". Increasing the blood pressure in this way promotes turbulent flow and increases the likelihood of fragments of tissue entering the blood stream on becoming detached from damaged vessels. During the morning surge, there is an increased risk of blood coagulation and of decreased fibrinolysis, both of which increase the risks posed by material that has detached from the vessel wall.

Increased risk of vessel obstruction during the morning surge is not predicted by monitoring ambulatory blood pressure over the previous 24 hours, nor by measurement of nocturnal BP levels nor by using scanners to detect asymptomatic stokes. The morning surge persists for 1-2 hours, at which time the risk of strokes and of coronary heart attacks is increased significantly. Hence, a morning surge constitutes a distinct risk factor for stroke and coronary heart attack and increased systolic pressure of 10 mm of mercury during the morning surge will increase the frequency of strokes by 22%. To counter this threat, drugs that lower blood pressure should be present in adequate amounts during the morning surge. Because of its early onset and the time needed for adequate absorption of tablets, anticipation is impractical. Avoiding a need for daily dosing is an effective solution. This can be achieved by using aliskiren, which inhibits the enzymatic action of renin. As only half of a dose is eliminated in 40 hours, adequate amounts of drug persist in circulating blood over 24 hours. As an alternative, daily dosing may be avoided by using a vaccine such as CZT0006, which induces formation of antibodies to neutralise effects of angiotensin II. As these antibodies are present in circulating blood for weeks or months, there is no need for daily dosing. By reducing blood pressure by 25 (systolic) and 13 (diastolic) mm of mercury, the early morning surge (between 0500 and 0800) can be nullified by CZT0006. Developments of this type illustrate how the increased knowledge of blood pressure control and of drug effects can progress beyond simple reduction of blood pressure.

4. Measuring blood pressure

4.1   Limitations of the mercury sphygmomanometer

- Using a sphygmomanometer requires training and expertise
- Subjective definition of the height of a column of mercury is biased towards prominent scale markings
- Errors arise due to poorly maintained sphygmomanometers and operators unfamiliar with the technical basis of measurement
- There is a significant risk from regular exposure to mercury vapour that escapes during use of the sphygmomanometer

Sphygmomanometers were used routinely throughout the last century. Hence, many adults and most clinicians will have some experience of this instrument. Such experience affects attitudes to measurement of blood pressure and has led to a resistance to replacement. Consequently, the merits of sphygmomanometers are overemphasised and they have been transmogrified from a useful clinical tool for measurement of blood pressure and have achieved the status of a "gold standard". The counterpart is an assertion that oscillometric self-measurement is inferior. In order to provide more balanced comparison, the merits and demerits of using sphygmomanometers have been reconsidered, even though these instruments cannot be used for self-measurement.

Specialised instruments provide precise and highly reproducible measurements of physical parameters. For instance, repeatedly weighing an inanimate object such as a brick on a spring balance will provide a series of identical readings. For corresponding parameters in animals there will be comparable consistency, as when measuring height and body weight. However, close inspection of replicate measurements of height and weight will reveal slight variation that becomes more pronounced if replicate measurements extend across the day. For body weight, this has an obvious explanation since the total water content will change continuously, with intake by intermittent eating and drinking being balanced by continuous loss due to respiration and perspiration as well as intermittent loss when voiding urine and faeces. Less obvious is the gradual compression of spinal constituents that causes a progressive, yet transient, reduction of height. Because such variation is inescapable, it is sensible to measure physical characteristics at a particular time and to spread replication over the day so that average values will be more representative of usual values. Replicated measurements of blood pressure vary from minute to minute, as well as within and between days. Hence, collection of replicated measurements will be needed for calculation of an average. The variation amongst replicated measurements of blood pressure can be considerable. To reduce the influence of unavoidable physical activity, as when standing or walking, it is recommended that subjects should remain seated and undisturbed for at least five minutes before self-measurement.

In the clinic, such an unhurried approach to measurement conflicts with the time constraints that govern a medical consultation. As consultation is likely to be limited to 10-15 minutes, the period of rest and relaxation will have to be foreshortened or, more probably, will be omitted. Hence, isolated measurements of blood pressure of uncertain precision are the rule rather than the exception, even though it is acknowledged that such lone measurements may fail to detect, or may erroneously indicate, high pressure. To avoid errors of this type, measurements have to be replicated and pooled so that an average can be calculated. During a medical consultation, such repetitive measurement is impracticable since the time needed would intrude into the time available for the next consultation. Hence, unless an initial measurement indicates elevated blood pressure, no additional measurements are likely; in effect, the infrastructure of medical consultation precludes precise measurement. As a compromise, the National Institute for Clinical Excellence (NICE) have recommended measurement of blood pressure at the onset of a consultation with repetition at the end of a consultation, but only if the initial measurement reveals a high pressure and only if sufficient time is available!

Replication of measurements with a mercury sphygmomanometer is time consuming because the undivided attention of a doctor or a trained medical assistant is needed to recognise the sounds that define systolic and diastolic pressures. After inflating a cuff around the upper arm, flow of blood into the forearm resumes as the cuff is slowly deflated. Systolic and diastolic pressures are defined by sounds within an artery that lies close to the inner surface of the elbow. Skill is needed to decide when these sounds indicate systolic and diastolic pressures whilst simultaneously assessing the height of a mercury column by eye from a scale adjacent to the column. Such division of attention predisposes to error and favours bias. As it is impracticable to attempt estimation of pressure to within 1 mm of mercury, the operator is likely to report particular terminal digits. This bias is easily revealed by inspection of replicate measurements which will typically reveal a disproportionate frequency of numbers ending with a zero (i.e. 120, 130 140 etc.) or with a five (i.e. 125, 135, 145 etc.). Such distortion is caused by the prominence of scale markings used to indicate measurement intervals and is legitimised by the pressures specified for lifestyle change (i.e. 115/75) and for diagnosis (i.e. 140/90). The resulting preference for particular terminal digits is not inconsequential. For instance, 140/90 is critical for treatment with drugs to lower blood pressure and misclassification could accelerate damage to vital organs. Such distortion can be offset by grouping measurements so that values ending in zero are dispersed centrally (i.e. 115-124, 125-134, 135-144 etc.).

During measurement of blood pressure with a sphygmomanometer, adherence to a protocol would minimise bias. Yet many who use these instruments lack the technical knowledge needed to make precise measurements and may be reluctant to adhere closely to a measurement protocol. Furthermore, procedural errors may be compounded by errors that stem from the instrument, which is not infrequent in sphygmomanometers that have not been serviced. For instance, inspection of approximately 500 mercury sphygmomanometers and their inflatable cuffs in use at a major teaching hospital in London revealed that more than half had defects that could cause significant inaccuracy. These deficiencies are overshadowed by the hazard posed by mercury. Properties that make mercury so well suited for pressure measurement in a sphygmomanometer make it difficult to contain. Leakage is not uncommon and, once spilled, mercury will be absorbed on contact with skin or when inhaled as an aerosol of fine droplets. Acute symptoms of toxicity are easy to avoid if mercury spillage is visible and can be contained in a fume cupboard. When there is no containment, chronic exposure to small amounts of mercury cannot be avoided. This hazard cannot be disregarded since such exposure to mercury may reduce fertility in women of childbearing age. Overall, limitations outweigh the merits of mercury sphygmomanometers and it is likely that mercury toxicity will be decisive when deciding whether these instruments should be abandoned (See Tables 9 & 10).

Almost universally accepted by doctors as a precise instrument
Robust
Does not require an electrical supply
Existing data that defines blood pressure as "high", "pre-hypertensive" or "normal" has largely been collected by using these instruments
Evidence relating frequency of strokes or coronary heart attacks to blood pressure has largely relied upon measurements with these instruments
Levels for introduction of lifestyle changes or of use of drugs to lower blood pressure have largely been determined by use of these instruments

Table 9. Merits of using a mercury sphygmomanometer

For reliable measurement, technical expertise is obligatory
Good ear to eye co-ordination is required to achieve precision
Preference for terminal digits ("5" or "0") contributes to imprecision
Meetings with an operator must be co-ordinated and may be cancelled
In 10-20% "masked hypertension" will remain undetected
In 20% "white coat effect" will cause significant overestimation
Replication of measurements is laborious and may be inconvenient
Chronic exposure to mercury vapour is likely

Table 10. Limitations of using a mercury sphygmomanometer

4.2 Use of semi-automated oscillometric manometers

- Measurement of blood pressure at hourly intervals over 24 hours will detect high blood pressure in ambulatory subjects
- Diurnal duplication of self-measurement over 7 days is a reliable alternative
- Pressures measured by semi-automated oscillometric manometers correspond closely with pressures measured by arterial cannulation
- Self-measurement avoids the apprehension and consequent error of measurements made in a clinic

Portable oscillometric manometers are used to record blood pressure in ambulatory patients. By keeping an inflatable cuff in place around the upper arm, it is possible to record measurements automatically at hourly intervals. Averaging such measurements over 24 hours is a reliable method for diagnosis of high blood pressure. As mercury sphygmomanometers cannot be used, in this way, automatic recording at hourly intervals only became feasible after oscillometric manometers had been accepted as a satisfactory method for measurement of blood pressure. Such ambulatory recording provides a major advance in blood pressure measurement, but wearing a cuff for 24 hours is discomforting. For this reason, regular self-measurement of blood pressure has been evaluated as an alternative that is less expensive and more readily accepted

Comparative studies have established that high blood pressure can be detected reliably by either method. Ambulatory measurements are more rapid, since recording is limited to 24 hours. For self-measurement, paired measurements of blood pressure are recorded each morning and evening and then averaged over seven days (i.e. 28 observations in total). Measurement with a mercury sphygmomanometer may achieve a comparable result if a nurse or doctor makes a pair of measurements during four separate visits to a clinic (i.e. 8 observations in total). These relatively large numbers of measurement sessions are needed because solitary measurements are unrepresentative. For instance, in a group of 150 ostensibly healthy individuals the incidence of high blood pressure was 40% by reference to these isolated measurements. Despite such imprecision, solitary measurements are preferred to prolongation of a medical consultation or to repeated visits to a clinic. Regular self-measurement at home with a semi-automatic oscillometric manometer is straightforward way of providing the replicates needed for calculation of averaged usual blood pressure. Although it is likely that isolated measurements will continue to be used during medical consultations, there is increasing awareness that self-measurement with semi-automatic oscillometric recorders could offer better blood pressure control.

Self-measurement is widely accepted for monitoring of body weight, blood glucose and lung function. It might be expected that self-measurement of usual blood pressure would similarly become a routine procedure. Exceptionally, there has been a reluctance to accept this methodology. For instance, in a recent review of blood pressure measurement it is asserted that "automated devices have been notorious for their inaccuracy" and that "the mercury manometer will have to be retained as a gold standard in designated laboratories". This opinion is pejorative since it links subjective assessment with "a gold standard" and "designated laboratories" yet describes objective recording as "notorious" and "inaccurate". It is irrational to discard automated measurement of blood pressure as inaccurate, since it is a technically impressive procedure of proven precision. For instance, by detecting a series of 12-15 heartbeats across the surface of the skin, blood pressures, pulse rate and radial artery waveforms can now be measured with a precision that matches corresponding measurements made with an indwelling arterial cannula. Transmogrifying the mercury sphygmomanometer to a "gold standard" is more akin to advertising than to science and dismissing all oscillometric manometers as "imprecise" is a generalisation that lacks foundation.

Usually, oscillometric measurement corresponds closely to measurements made by a sphygmomanometer or an electronic pressure transducer linked to an intra-arterial cannula. If slight differences are detected, these will be inconsequential if compared with the rise of pressure that many individuals experience on entry into clinical surroundings. Apprehension of measurement on entering medical surroundings causes the "white coat effect", when measurements of systolic blood pressure may exceed usual blood pressure by 10-20 mm of mercury or more. Such overestimation eclipses possible instrumentation error by an order of magnitude. When medical or paramedical staff measure blood pressure within the confines of a clinic this type of error is unavoidable and self-measurement is the only way to circumvent this limitation. As self-measurement has been increasingly used in recent years finding of even greater significance has emerged. It is now apparent that between 10 and 20% of individuals whose blood pressure appears to be normal in the clinic will have high blood pressure that can be detected by self-measurement. This "masked hypertension" is associated with an increased risk of damage to target organs that is not dissimilar to the increased risk of patients whose blood pressure is high when measured in the clinic. Without self-measurement, these individuals would, in effect, experience high blood pressure without treatment.

When using the oscillometric method for measurement of blood pressure, systolic and diastolic pressures are inferred from a group of successive pressure changes. These indirect measurements can be validated by comparison with contemporaneous measurements from a cannula placed within an artery. Veterinarians used this strategy to validate oscillometric measurement of blood pressure in dogs. By placing a cuff at the base of the tail, it is possible to demonstrate that replicate oscillometric measurements reflect arterial pressures measured directly from within an artery. Such comparisons between indirect and direct measurement are rarely practicable in healthy individuals since arterial cannulation is an invasive procedure that produces discomfort. Moreover, use of arterial cannulation for instrument evaluation would be considered to be unethical since the outcome could be predicted from results in experimental animals. Hence, arterial cannulation is rarely used to validate precision of semi-automatic oscillometric instruments. Instead, certification of precision for semi-automatic oscillometric recorders relies upon comparison between pressure measurements obtained by semi-automatic oscillometry and contemporaneous measurement using mercury manometry, both in subjects with normal blood pressure and in patients with high blood pressure. The American Association for the Advancement of Medical Instrumentation and the British Hypertension Society use this approach to evaluate specific instruments. Oscillometers are deemed to be acceptable if averaged pressures are matched by mercury sphygmomanometers. Relying upon mercury sphygmomanometers to provide an absolute level of precision is convenient. However, pressures from an indwelling cannula provide a more rigorous test. In one such comparison, over three hundred measurements from indwelling arterial cannulae were compared with automated oscillometric measurements in the contralateral arm. Correlation was close (ratio 0.96) and the difference between measurements of systolic pressure by the two methods never exceeded 5 mm of mercury.

Semi-automatic oscillometric recording is convenient for monitoring patients with high blood pressure (systolic >140 mm of mercury or diastolic >90 mm of mercury) or individuals at risk of progressing to high blood pressure (systolic pressure >115 mm of mercury or diastolic pressure >75 mm of mercury). However, there are circumstances for which oscillometic recording may not be appropriate. For instance, pressures recorded by mercury manometers in pregnancy will not match measurements from all types of oscillometric recorders. For self-measurement of blood pressure in pregnancy, it is therefore important to select an electronic oscillometric recorder that has been approved specifically for this condition (e.g. Omron-MIT, Omron Elite 7300W, Microlife 3BTO-A(2) or Microlife WatchBP Home). Similarly, when patients have abnormal heart rhythm, pressures measured using a mercury sphygmomanometer may not correspond to pressures measured using electronic oscillometry. It is important therefore to establish that your own medical history does not preclude self-measurement by semi-automatic oscillometry. It may be presumed that use of such instruments will be appropriate for most patients with high blood pressure and for healthy individuals who have not yet progressed to high blood pressure. Moreover, because of the problems posed by the "white coat" effect and the limitations of solitary or intermittent measurements, it is reasonable to presume that self-measurements will frequently be more precise than intermittent measurement in a clinic. Indeed, for the 10-20% of unselected subjects who have masked hypertension, self-measurement may be their only hope.

Overall, the advantages of semi-automatic oscillometry for self-measurement of blood pressure greatly outweigh its disadvantages (See Tables 11 & 12). With recognition of the importance of raised blood pressure as a cause of organ damage during pre-hypertension, it can be expected that self-measurement will be used increasingly in prevention, as well as during treatment, of high blood pressure.

Objective measurement with a digital display
Semi-automatic measurement does not require expertise
Replication of measurements is rapid and easy
Ease of regular measurement allows trend detection
Can be used at home, at work and when travelling
Detects "masked hypertension"
Unaffected by the "white coat effect"

Table 11. Advantages of semi-automatic oscillometric measurement of blood pressure

Replication over 7 days needed for reliable estimation of usual blood pressure
Self-measurements may be falsified
Imprecision increases with increased stiffening of the arteries
Irregular heartbeats may lead to imprecise estimation of usual blood pressure
May not be suitable for pregnancy

Table 12. Disadvantages of semi-automatic oscillometric measurement of blood pressure

4.3   A need for multiple estimates of blood pressures

- Hourly measurements over a period of 24 hours give an average that matches usual blood pressure
- Isolated measurements of blood pressure often fail to match the average of several measurements
- When measured in a clinic, averaged blood pressure is calculated from paired observations recorded on four separate occasions
- When measured at home, averaged blood pressure is calculated from paired observations made twice daily over seven days

Regular measurements reveal that normal blood pressure changes little month by month (See Figure 17). Since isolated measurements vary substantially throughout a single day and between separate days, this stability of usual blood pressure is impressive (See Table 13 & Figure 18). Nevertheless, measurement of blood pressure on a single day cannot be relied upon to indicate usual blood pressure since pressure can vary by as much as 20 (systolic) mm of mercury (See Figure 19). Some sources of this wide variation are known and understood. For instance, blood pressure is liable to rise following physical activity and during periods of stress; conversely, blood pressure will fall during inactivity, as after a meal or during sleep. It is not therefore unexpected that there will be variation, even when a fixed time for measurement has been selected. Because of the considerable variation between and within individual days, isolated measurements do not necessarily indicate usual blood pressure and may be misleading. For this reason, a systolic blood pressure of 140 mm of mercury will be overestimated (at more than 165 mm of mercury) and underestimated (at less than 115 mm of mercury) once in every twenty measurements. A similar degree of variation occurs in those individuals who are pre-hypertensive and, with a systolic blood pressure of 130 mm of mercury. In such individuals, measurement of systolic blood pressure can be expected to exceed 140 mm of mercury or to be less than 120 mm of mercury, once in every in every six occasions. The prospect of arriving at conclusions that are diametrically opposed (i.e. high blood pressure at 140 mm of mercury or optimal blood pressure at 120 mm of mercury) reveals why it is not possible to use isolated measurements either for diagnosis or for control during treatment.

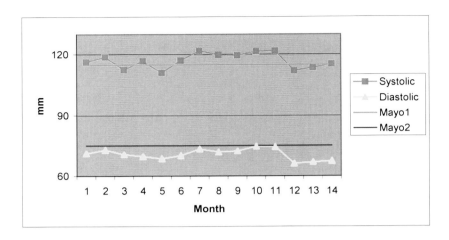

Figure 17. Consistency of monthly measurements (March-April) of usual systolic blood pressure.

The nature of this problem is illustrated by 216 sequential self-measurements recorded daily at 0900, 1500 & 2100 hrs. The averaged systolic pressure from this group of measurements is 132 mm of mercury, which is not dissimilar from averages for this individual in previous months. Although there is month-on-month consistency, the individual measurements of systolic pressure that determine this average of 132 range between 97 and 157 mm of mercury. No particular measurement predominates. On 10 occasions, the systolic pressure was 136 mm of mercury; yet on eight occasions it was 119, 122, 123, 124, 127, 131, 132, 133 & 144 mm of mercury.

Systolic pressure (mm of mercury)						
95 (0)	105 (2)	115 (0)	125 (6)	135 (5)	145 (6)	155 (1)
96 (0)	106 (1)	116 (5)	126 (5)	136 (10)	146 (5)	156 (1)
97 (1)	107 (1)	117 (4)	127 (8)	137 (3)	147 (3)	157 (1)
98 (0)	108 (1)	118 (3)	128 (5)	138 (4)	148 (1)	158 (0)
99 (0)	109 (3)	119 (8)	129 (4)	139 (6)	149 (2)	159 (0)
100 (1)	110 (3)	120 (6)	130 (3)	140 (3)	150 (1)	160 (0)
101 (0)	111 (5)	121 (3)	131 (8)	141 (2)	151 (2)	161 (0)
102 (0)	112 (3)	122 (9)	132 (8)	142 (2)	152 (5)	162 (0)
103 (0)	113 (4)	123 (8)	133 (8)	143 (6)	153 (2)	163 (0)
104 (0)	114 (4)	124 (8)	134 (4)	144 (8)	154 (3)	164 (0)

Table 13. Frequency (in brackets) of individual measurements of systolic blood pressure within a sequence of 216 successive measurements made in a single subject whilst at rest

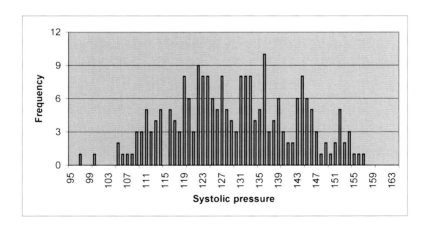

Figure 18. Distribution of a series of 216 successive measurements from a single individual.

It is of interest to determine whether averaging measurements for a single day might provide an acceptable estimate. Averaging measurements for a single day curtails variation. Most averages lie between 131 and 135 mm of mercury and hence approximate to the monthly average of 132 mm of mercury. Even so, the range extends from 118 to 144 mm of mercury (See Figure 19) and, as daily averages can differ by as much as 26 mm of mercury, they do not give a satisfactory indication of usual blood pressure (See Figure 19). To estimate usual blood pressure with adequate precision, several daily measurements must be pooled. A practical consequence is that relatively large numbers of regular measurements are needed to detect significant effects when lifestyle is changed or when there is changed drug treatment. Attempting to detect a trend towards high blood pressure will require replicate measurements over a long period and will demand close adherence to a measurement protocol.

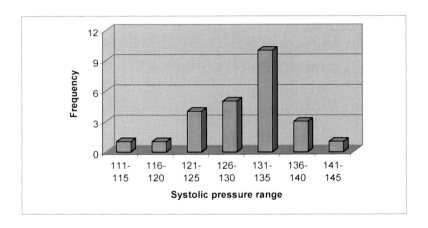

Figure 19. Averaged daily measurements calculated from a series of 216 successive measurements (mean 132 mm of mercury) in a single individual.

On the basis of studies in large numbers of patients, a protocol has been recommended for detection of high blood pressure from measurements made in a clinic. Using four separate visits to provide paired measurements at each visit will give a total of eight measurements that can be averaged to provide an acceptable estimate of usual blood pressure. Such averages are recommended for diagnosis. The same procedure should also be used to decide whether treatment is satisfactory by comparing averaged pressure during treatment with averaged pressure before treatment. It follows that a minimum of four visits to the clinic would be needed to establish a baseline for comparison with the levels detected during further grouped visits. Because of the high prevalence of high blood pressure in developed countries, it is impracticable to contemplate such a cumbersome procedure. If every patient with high blood pressure had to make a minimum of eight successive visits on separate days for assessment of blood pressure control, clinics and their staff would be overwhelmed. For this reason, intermittent isolated measurements continue to be used routinely to assess blood pressure control, even though it is widely acknowledged that the method is fundamentally flawed.

Self-measurement of blood pressure offers a simple solution to the problem of making regular measurements in these very large numbers of individuals. It enables blood pressure to be closely controlled during treatment and, furthermore, is the only realistic approach for detection of transition from normal to pre-hypertension and progression from pre-hypertension to high blood pressure. This form of monitoring has the advantage over clinical measurement of detecting masked hypertension, which will occur in more than one out of ten with high blood pressure, and avoids the problem of white coat hypertension, which occurs in more than one in five of the remainder. Although self-measurement can indicate the onset of high blood pressure, such diagnosis would have to be confirmed by a doctor. Once high blood pressure has been recognised, there can be no reconsideration. Of greater interest to the patient is access to a method that will detect loss of blood pressure control during treatment. Because of the ease of self-measurement, recording duplicate measurements each morning and evening for seven successive days need not be an inconvenience, especially if compared with the alternative of multiple visits to a clinic. The protocol for self-measurement yields 28 measurements that can be pooled to provide averaged blood pressure each week with a precision that matches, or exceeds, the average derived from replicate clinical measurements obtained during four separate visits to a clinic. If widely used to avoid high blood pressure, self-measurement could rank with vaccination or mass screening by X-rays as a public health measure.

4.4   Using self-measurement to make decisions

- An average of self-measurements over one week can be used for diagnosis of high blood pressure
- Averages of weekly measurements will confirm whether treatment by drugs is adequate
- Averages of weekly measurements will detect whether exercise, changed diet, reduced body weight or use of alternative therapies reduces blood pressure appreciably
- Over long periods, regular or intermittent weekly measurements will detect any upward trend of blood pressure

Solitary measurements of blood pressure are useful whenever exceptionally high pressures are detected, since it is mandatory to give prompt medical attention if blood pressures exceed 180 (systolic) or 130 (diastolic) mm of mercury. On making such a finding, it would be prudent to repeat the measurement after resting and relaxing, so that the exceptional nature of the measurement can be confirmed unequivocally. More usually, it will not be possible to make any conclusion from an isolated measurement, excepting that further measurements would be needed to confirm, or exclude, high blood pressure. Should high blood pressure be recognised, there will be a need for treatment. Almost invariably this will cause drugs to be prescribed and it is highly likely that a changed lifestyle would also be recommended. It may be recalled that regular weekly measurements are needed to confirm that treatment is adequate since isolated measurements cannot achieve this objective and since even replicate measurements made within a single day can be misleading (See Figures 18 & 19).

Deciding whether or not blood pressure is high enough to require treatment is a decision that will be made by your doctor. In general, it can be expected that pressures in excess of 140 (systolic) or 90 (diastolic) mm of mercury will prompt an introduction of drugs to lower blood pressure because these pressures are associated with unacceptable risks of stroke or coronary heart attack. There is some room for some flexibility in elderly patients, for whom a threshold of 160 mm of mercury for systolic pressure merits consideration (See Figure 14).

Although it is relatively straightforward to set targets for introduction of treatment, setting targets for control of blood pressure during treatment is more difficult. By monitoring very large numbers of individuals, it can be establishes that death rate from strokes or coronary heart attacks are proportional to usual blood pressure (See Figures 2, 3 & 4). The risk of strokes and coronary heart attacks rises progressively as usual blood pressure rises, but it cannot be presumed that these risks during treatment must decline at the same rate during treatment. Hence, although target pressures as low as 115 (systolic) and 75 (diastolic) mm of mercury might be considered, it has not been established that there is a proportionate reduced risk as pressures fall below 140 (systolic) and 90 (diastolic) mm of mercury. Furthermore, it has to be taken on trust that any risk reduction will be uniformly continuous as blood pressure falls and will not take the form of a plateau.

The "Hypertension Optimal Treatment Study" was devised specifically to resolve this issue. By correlating the frequency of strokes and coronary heart attacks with the level of blood pressure during treatment, it is possible to specify usual blood pressures that should not be exceeded whilst patients are being treated. In this study, pressures in excess of 138.5 (systolic) or 82.6 (diastolic) mm of mercury were associated with a progressive increase in the frequency of strokes and coronary heart attacks in this study yet further reduction afforded no additional protection. These pressures do not differ markedly from the target levels of 140 (systolic) and 85 (diastolic) mm of mercury set by the British Hypertensive Society.

The "Cardio-Sis" study has addressed a complementary question when the target for reduced systolic blood pressure was set below 130 rather than the usual target of 140 mm of mercury. Within two years of starting tighter control of systolic pressure, the incidence of left ventricular hypertrophy was 11%, which is a substantial improvement on the 17% incidence when adopting conventional control. Such it could be expected that diminished ventricular damage would limit untoward cardiovascular events and these were halved during this period of tight control.

Whether target systolic pressure lower than 130 mm of mercury will offer additional benefit has yet to be investigated. Although, in effect, this policy of

113

target reduction has been adopted to avoid strokes and coronary heart attacks in diabetic patients, when target pressures are set at 130 (systolic) and 80 (diastolic) mm of mercury or even lower. In diabetic patients, the extent and intensity of damage to arterial vessels is predicted by the usual concentration of glucose in plasma. Hence, poor control of blood glucose will make diabetic patients especially vulnerable to the surges of pressure that precipitate strokes or coronary heart attacks. In diabetic patients, these risks can be increased even when concentrations of glucose in plasma lie within the normal range. It is therefore possible that vessel damage resulting from diabetes contributes to morbidity and mortality more than expected. In this context, it should be noted that subtle deficiencies of blood glucose control are detectable in many, and possibly most, patients with high blood pressure. It is therefore possible that empirical reduction of blood pressure without limitation might increase protection of arteries and reduce the overall incidence of strokes and coronary heart attacks in other sub-groups as well as in diabetics.

When usual blood pressure exceeds thresholds of 115 (systolic) or 75 (diastolic) mm of mercury, the risk of strokes and coronary heart attacks rises and the risk increases, regardless of whether subjects are ostensibly healthy or are being treated for high blood pressure (See Figures 2, 3 & 4). It is tempting to presume that these risks will fall in a comparable manner as blood pressure is lowered. Yet the existence of a threshold below which reducing usual blood pressure offers no further protection suggests that it may not be possible to reverse all of the vessel damage that underlies an increased risk of strokes and heart attacks.

In experimental animals, prolonged exposure of arterial vessels to raised blood pressure will stimulate growth of arterial muscle. These structural changes closely resemble those in the vessels of patients with longstanding high blood pressure. Such structural changes could contribute to the increased risk of strokes and coronary heart. In such circumstances, drugs that relax arterial muscle or promote excretion of sodium cannot be expected to influence this risk factor. Other structural changes that are also irreversible can make a similar contribution. For instance, prolonged exposure to raised blood pressure can produce irretrievable damage individual filtration units in the kidney. As loss of damaged filtration units is cumulative, elimination of sodium and water will diminish progressively. It is therefore to be expected that elevation of blood pressure for a long period will increase the risk of strokes and coronary heart attacks. This residual risk can be emphasised by using a "logistic spline plot" to display these risks and the increase with age implies that the damage is irreversible (See Figures 12,13 & 14). A residual risk of strokes and coronary heart attacks is apparent even when blood pressures are less than 115 (systolic) or 75 (diastolic) mm of mercury and this may constitute a plateau of the type revealed in logistic spline plots. This would make intelligible the persistence of risk below thresholds of 115 (systolic) or 75 (diastolic) mm of mercury and yet be consistent with the absence of stokes and coronary heart attacks in non-acculturated communities.

Blood pressure measurements vary both within and between days. Hence, they must be averaged over a period of time to define usual blood pressure with any certainty. Measurement over one week should suffice to reveal whether pressures of 140 (systolic) and 90 (diastolic) mm of mercury are being exceeded. However, recording pressures over several weeks will be needed to assess effects of changed lifestyle (e.g. exercise, diet, changed BMI or use of alternative therapies) because incremental pressure changes are often small and may be slow to develop. Longer periods of observation are also needed to decide whether lowering of blood pressure during treatment is adequate. For instance, withdrawal of a diuretic drug may continue to cause increased arterial pressure for several weeks. Hence, when defining a baseline for usual blood pressure, it is sensible to use a series of weekly measurements since a larger number of measurements will increase the likelihood that your estimate of usual blood pressure is valid. Reliably establishing usual blood pressure with series of weekly measurements will greatly facilitate testing for idiosyncratic sensitivity to substances (e.g. salt) or effects of factors that may vary over time (e.g. stress).

Weekly measurements that have been collected over longer periods will reveal any progression towards high blood pressure. As arterial damage is cumulative and slow to develop, there may be a window of opportunity to pre-empt such damage. It is difficult to estimate the duration of high pressure needed to induce irreversible arterial damage. Since the high blood pressure of pregnancy can be reversed fully, it is possible that several months may be needed for changes to become irreversible. In light of this, it would be prudent for young people to make intermittent measurement of blood pressure (e.g. at intervals of three or six months) to provide a platform that will aid detection of any upward trend. It might be noted that this would require much less time and effort than undertaking regular tests of vision or dental heath and would have the advantage over these other types of routine tests of offering substantial prolongation of life. For individuals who have already become pre-hypertensive, more frequent measurement is advisable to detect continuation of the upward trend and to establish whether attempting lifestyle changes (e.g. increased aerobic exercise, reduced body weight) is effective. For patients with high blood pressure, regular monitoring is obligatory to confirm that adequate treatment is being used since any increase of blood pressure above 135 (systolic) or 80 (diastolic) mm of mercury will increase the risk of disability or death due to strokes or coronary heart attacks.

5. Recording your measurements

- Avoid recent exertion to ensure that you will be relaxed
- Make your measurements under the same conditions and at the same time of day
- Estimate usual blood pressure by averaging successive replicate measurements
- If being treated for high blood pressure, record your blood pressure over several days prior to medical consultation
- If not already affected by high blood pressure, use averaged self-measurements to guard against an upward trend

Physical activity results in an increase of blood pressure that can persist for many minutes. Hence, an initial self-measurement in a series of replicates will often overestimate usual blood pressure. Obviously, you should not engage in vigorous physical activity before self-measurement and you should be alert to the possibility of residual effects of earlier activities. Before commencing self-measurement, you should be seated comfortably and should have relaxed for at least five minutes. This will reduce variation between replicate measurements and helps to avoid inclusion of unrepresentative measurements when calculating averaged blood pressure. The timing of regular measurements should be set to fit with your lifestyle. Arbitrary times of 0900 & 1800 used throughout but other fixed times in the morning or evening might be more convenient. Whatever times are used, variation in timing should be avoided since diurnal changes due to hormone secretion are inflexible and, like feeding and bathing, could introduce bias.

The problem posed by physical activity is illustrated by a succession of self-measurements recorded immediately after completing some domestic cleaning (See Table 14). The first measurement was made without delay and was immediately followed by successive measurements at intervals of approximately 90 seconds, the time required to complete and record each measurement. In the first measurement of the series, systolic and diastolic pressures were high and the pulse rate raised by comparison with subsequent measurements. These values, together with those from the second and third measurements, imply that recovery from the activity was incomplete. Over the preceding 30 days, daily self-measurement had established that usual systolic blood pressure was 130 mm of mercury. In the present series, systolic blood pressure did not approach this level until the fourth measurement. In effect therefore, these first three measurements have occupied the five minute period that should have been allocated to rest and recovery. In subsequent measurements, there was no obvious trend and an average from the fourth to the tenth measurement (131 mm of mercury) did not deviate appreciably from usual systolic blood pressure (130 mm of mercury).

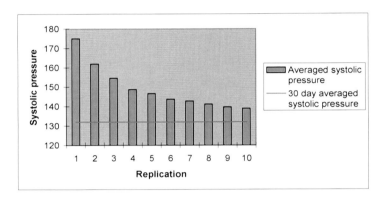

Figure 20. Systolic pressures averaged by grouping successive measurements (1, 1+2, 1+2+3, etc.) exceed the averaged systolic pressure over the preceding 30 days.

Rank Order	Blood pressure (mm of mercury)		Pulse rate (beats/min)
	Systolic	Diastolic	
1	175	101	56
2	149	94	50
3	140	94	46
4	131	89	48
5	138	89	48
6	129	89	46
7	137	80	45
8	130	81	47
9	128	85	43
10	132	85	44

Table 14. Replicate measurements of systolic and diastolic blood pressures together with pulse rates in a single subject over a period of approximately 15 minutes.

This series of measurements demonstrates how omission of a period of rest and relaxation can lead to imprecision. Initial measurement of systolic pressure is 175 mm of mercury and inclusion of this value when calculating averages has a disproportionate influence. For instance, 162 mm of mercury is the average of the first two measurements of systolic pressure and 155 mm of mercury the average of the first three measurements. Even an average of all ten replicates (139) is differs substantially from the averaged daily measurement (132.0) over the preceding 30 days (See Figure 20). Error largely arises because the first three measurements in the series. These substantially exceed the monthly average whereas the remaining six measurements (fourth to the tenth replicates) give an average (131.5) that is close to the pressure measured over the previous thirty days (132.0).

It is impracticable to exclude all activities in a domestic environment as a prelude to self-measurement. Sitting at rest for five minutes with a cuffed arm supported by a cushion or pillow therefore can serve as a compromise with the advantage of becoming a routine part of each measurement session. Five minutes may seem inconsequential; yet, even this brief period of compulsory inactivity can be frustrating. It is fortunate that background music or viewing light entertainment on a television does not introduce variation. For this reason, a seat that is used habitually to view television or to listen to music may facilitate relaxation. Because only a few minutes are needed for self-measurement, it may be tempting to make changes. However, changes are likely to introduce error. In seating that is unfamiliar, relaxation may be hampered by conscious, or subconscious, tension in muscles of the trunk and legs and by contractions of muscles in the arms or shoulders. It is important to avoid restlessness or even conscious suppression of such movements, as well as coughing, speaking or sitting crossed legged. Not surprisingly, either making or anticipating a visit to the toilet immediately prior to self-measurement would bias measurements. By the same token, it is necessary to exclude recent consumption of drinks (tea, coffee, cola, alcoholic beverages), smoking and exposure to heat or cold (e.g. taking a bath or shower or returning indoors from hot, cold or wet conditions). Sudden disturbance (e.g. unexpected noise) will cause a surge of pressure as also will arrival, or even anticipation, of incoming telephone calls. To ensure that indirect measurements of blood pressure match pressure in the large arteries, the detector on the cuff must be positioned at the level of the heart. This can be achieved by supporting the arm upon a cushion, which will help the muscles of the arm and shoulder to relax.

In a sequence of self-measurements of blood pressure, it is not unusual for the first measurement to be appreciably higher than subsequent measurements. Such overestimation may merely indicate an insufficient period of rest and relaxation (See Table 14, Figure 20). On the other hand, it may be an inevitable feature of such serial measurements (See Figure 21). For instance, the cuff is likely to become slightly repositioned after an initial inflation and re-inflation and this will influence perception and reduce apprehension. As in "white coat hypertension", individuals may be apprehensive of the measurement procedure or its outcome. It will not be possible to eliminate all such factors, excepting by excluding initial measurements. Discarding the first measurement can provide a pragmatic solution when calculating averaged blood pressures and is a pre-defined feature of at least one model of semi-automatic oscillometer.

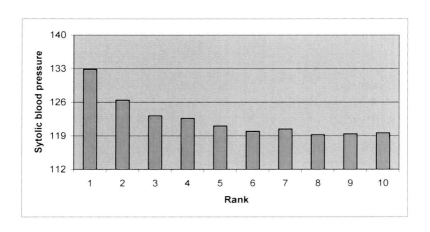

Figure 21. Effect of rank order of measurement upon averaged systolic blood pressure illustrated by pooling measurements from 100 successive sessions, each with ten-fold replication

By placing a cuff at the base of the tail, blood pressure can be measured in dogs in a manner that corresponds to measurements in humans. Between four and six-fold replication will give averages that correspond to measurements taken from a cannula within a large artery. Comparable replication should be satisfactory in humans. The interval between multiple measurements does not influence precision since, by using a specially modified instrument, it has been shown that an interval of 15 seconds between measurements does not influence accuracy. Since a single measurement can be completed and recorded within one and a half minutes, regular measurements may be repeated as quickly as is practicable. This would allow three successive self-measurements to be completed within five minutes. The official recommendation for self-measurement of blood pressure is to make paired measurements at each session. Using more replicates will improve precision, but will prolong the measurement session. For instance, recording four rather than two sequential measurements would prolong each measurement session by three minutes and extend the measurement session from eight (i.e. 5 + 3) minutes to eleven (i.e. 5 + 6) minutes. This is a modest increase and prolongation of the measurement session may be preferred since improved precision is complemented by a need for less frequent measurement sessions, especially when monitoring long-term trends.

6. Selecting an option for self-measurement

- **Option one**: calculation of averaged blood pressures from duplicate measurements made morning and evening for seven successive days
- **Option two**: calculation of averaged blood pressures from triplicate measurements made morning and evening for seven successive days, after discarding the initial measurement from each triplicate
- **Option three**: calculation of averaged blood pressures from quadruplicate measurements made morning and evening for seven successive days, after discarding the initial measurement from each quadruplicate
- **Option four**: monitoring usual blood pressures using weekly averaged pressures
- **Option five**: recording averaged pressures before and after changing treatment

Measurements of blood pressure will vary considerably from day to day. Hence, it is exceptional for isolated measurements to match measurements that have been averaged. In order to measure usual blood pressure, a group of individual measurements have to be averaged by following a procedure specified in "The International Consensus Conference on Self-Measurement of Blood Pressure". This stipulates that two measurements should be made at a fixed time each morning and evening for seven successive days. These twenty-eight measurements are pooled in order to calculate an average of usual blood pressure.

Despite using twenty-eight measurements, it is nevertheless likely that usual blood pressure will be overestimated. This error arises because the first measurement of a series of blood pressure measurements is likely to be the highest. For instance, the paired measurements that comprise Figure 22 average 137 for the initial measurements and 128 for the final measurements. Hence, inclusion of the initial measurements inclines towards overestimation. With small numbers of measurements this bias may not be obvious. With larger numbers of measurements, bias is readily revealed when measurements are averaged according to rank order, as in Figure 21. Averaged initial measurements exceed averaged measurements from the second rank; in turn, averaged measurements from the second rank exceed averaged measurements from the third rank. Effects of rank order only become insignificant from the fifth or sixth replicates and beyond. In biology, such variation is not uncommon. Hence, triplicate or quadruplicate measurements are commonplace in laboratory experiments. This level of replication not only allows for variation but also detects unrepresentative measurements that are possibly unsound for technical reasons. It may be recalled that when direct and indirect measurements of blood pressure were compared in the dog, an average of four replicates of the indirect measurements were needed to match direct measurement from an intra-arterial cannula.

Because of the effect of rank order, it is preferable to make more than the recommended paired measurements of blood pressure at each session. More replication will prolong the measurement session but will increase the precision of estimated blood pressure. As much of the error associated with replication can be attributed to the first measurement, discarding these initial measurements might achieve a more acceptable level of precision. To provide the 28 measurements needed for calculation of usual blood pressure, three-fold replication would be needed. Using four-fold replication will yield an average that is an even more reliable estimate of usual blood pressure.

Much emphasis has been given to the precision of instruments used for measurement of blood pressure. Yet, it should be recognised that variations arising during the measurement procedure will overshadow errors that stem from the measuring instruments. As has already been pointed out, recent physical exertion will distort averaged blood pressure (See Figure 20). Detecting and reducing this type of error is relatively straightforward, although elimination is difficult. Such a decline may be revealed if individuals experience a "white coat effect" on entering a medical environment. Their apprehension will cause overestimation of systolic pressure by 20 mm of mercury or more and can be revealed by making successive self-measurements, whilst in isolation. As well as detecting a "white coat" effect, this procedure incidentally illustrates the progressive decline of blood pressure with increased replication.

During self-measurement, there is therefore a trade-off between increased precision and prolongation of measurement sessions. Greater replication increases the precision of averaged measurements of blood pressure but inescapably prolongs each measurement session. Even so, prolongation of a measurement session by a few minutes might well be attractive to those who are using self-measurement intermittently. This is because the higher precision that results from increased replication within an individual measurement session could justify less frequent measurement sessions. An individual who is monitoring usual blood pressures three or four times a year in order to detect any slight upward trend might well favour a prolongation of a measurement session to be sure of greater precision. Whichever method is selected, graphical display of measurements is recommended since plotted data be assimilated very quickly by clinicians and will justify the average that you cite for your usual blood pressure.

As you accumulate measurements, you will begin to appreciate why these measurements are essential for detection of deterioration of blood pressure control. In this respect, control of blood pressure is quite different from control of body mass. When measuring body mass, bathroom scales are helpful, but are not essential. Changed body weight is indicated by your image in a mirror, the fit of your clothes and the comments of your family and friends. Readings from the bathroom scales merely reinforce what is already obvious. Moreover, the deterioration of heath that arises in individuals who are overweight is, in large part, readily reversed by weight reduction. High blood pressure cannot be perceived in this way and clandestine tissue damage is, in large part irreversible and will not be revealed until severe symptoms arise suddenly and without warning, as during a stroke or a coronary heart attack. Regular self-measurement of blood pressure should therefore be considered obligatory rather than optional.

As self-measurement sessions need to be undertaken in comfort, the method selected for transcribing measurements should be simple and convenient. Some blood pressure monitors accumulate measurements for later recall. Preferably, a portable electronic device should be used to record measurements as they arise, as when using an app on a smart phone. If being noted on paper, a notebook is strongly recommended in order to avoid confusion and data loss when measurements are entered into a computer at a later date.

OPTION ONE

Determination of usual blood pressure

In accord with "The International Consensus Conference on Self Blood Pressure Measurement" usual blood pressures is determined by making duplicate measurements each morning and evening for seven days in succession. Measurements are made at the same time each day (e.g. 0900 and 1800) and averaged usual blood pressure is calculated by using all of the 28 measurements.

OPTION TWO

Determination of usual blood pressure

To reduce bias due to the initial measurement, three measurements are made each morning and each evening for seven successive days. For calculation of averaged blood pressure, only the second and third measurements from each group of three sequential measurements are used. Hence, averaged usual blood pressure is calculated by using 28 of the 42 measurements.

OPTION THREE

Determination of usual blood pressure

To reduce bias due to the initial measurement and to provide greater precision, four measurements are made each morning and each evening for seven successive days. For calculation of averaged blood pressure, only the second, third and fourth measurements are used. Hence, averaged usual blood pressure is calculated by using 42 of the 56 measurements.

OPTION FOUR

Long term monitoring of blood pressure

Irrespective of the option selected for measurement of usual blood pressure and whether such measurements are made intermittently or regularly, averages are plotted on an annual scale (52 weeks). If being treated for high blood pressure, a graphical presentation of these averaged pressures provides a simple and convenient way of indicating satisfactory control. As well as being useful for monitoring control, the same method can be used to detect the upward trend that is a precursor of pre-hypertension.

OPTION FIVE

Detecting the effect of changed treatment

In order to assess the effect on blood pressure of any treatment or change of treatment, it is necessary to make comparison with earlier measurements. The act of diagnosis provides a body of measurements against which effects of treatment can be gauged. For high blood pressure of longstanding, measurements can be made in anticipation of any changed treatment. If you have not been making measurements routinely, you should recommence regular measurement for at least a week before a change of treatment. Obviously, regular measurement should become a routine if there has been a need for changed treatment.

Comparison between two groups of measurements is a sensitive method for detecting changes when drugs are being introduced or withdrawn or when the dose of a drug is being changed. It is also possible to use such paired comparisons to detect effects of particular activities, such as exercise, diet or work. For instance, measurements of blood pressures during weekends can be compared with measurements during an equal number of working days. By this means, the effect of increased exercise or intense physical work can be compared periods of relative inactivity. A similar comparison between a period at work or on vacation may detect an effect of stress on usual blood pressure.

7. Representative examples

Self-measurement is used to monitor blood pressure when normal and healthy, when pre-hypertensive and when high blood pressure has been recently recognised or is long established and possibly poorly controlled. In all of these circumstances, the methods used for recording and presenting measurements is the same, excepting that individuals who are normal or pre-hypertensive will be likely to make measurements less frequently. Examples that have been chosen depict measurements during the phase of pre-hypertension (Options 1-3), whilst approaching pre-hypertension (Option 4) and during treatment of high blood pressure (Option 5).

To provide a common body of data for the first three of these examples, four successive measurements of blood pressure were recorded each morning and each evening for seven successive days. By this means, a common group of measurements can illustrate differences between options one, two and three (See Figures 22, 23 and 24).

OPTION ONE

By using the only first two measurements from each group, averaged blood pressure can be calculated using option one. Figure 22 shows how the averaged systolic pressure changed between morning and evening sessions for seven successive days and a horizontal line depicts the averaged pressure for that week. It is noticeable that only on day five are the morning and evening measurements close to the average measurement for the week.

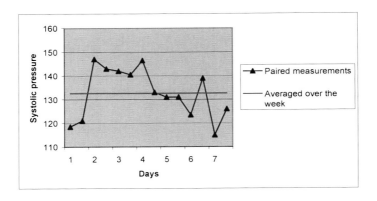

Figure 22. Calculation of average systolic blood pressure from twenty-eight measurements collected over seven days.

OPTION TWO

By using the second and third measurements from each group, averaged blood pressure can be calculated for option two (i.e. discarding the first of triplicate measurements). Figure 23 shows how the averaged systolic pressure changed between morning and evening sessions for seven successive days includes a horizontal line that depicts averaged pressure for that week. Only in the morning of day five and in the evenings in days three, five and six are these measurements close to the average for the week. The average for the week using option two is lower than the average obtained by use of paired measurements in option one and illustrates how exclusion of initial measurements can appreciably reduce estimated blood pressure.

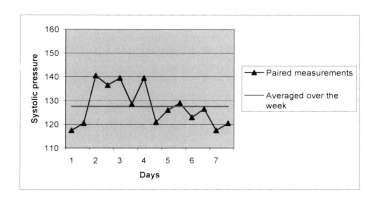

Figure 23. Calculation of average systolic blood pressure from twenty-eight of forty-two measurements collected over seven days.

OPTION THREE

By using the second, third and fourth measurements from each group, averaged blood pressure can be calculated as for option three (i.e. discarding the first of quadruplicate measurements). Figure 24 shows how the averaged systolic pressure changed between morning and evening sessions for seven successive days and includes a horizontal line that depicts averaged pressure for that week. Averaged measurements are only very close to the average for the week on the evening of day six.

When paired measurements of blood pressure are used to calculate averaged pressure by option one, variation of day to day pressure is greater than for the other two options. Omission of the first measurement also reduces variation in option three and further reduced the range of variation. As anticipated, weekly average pressures calculated by option one are higher than weekly averages calculated when using options two or three.

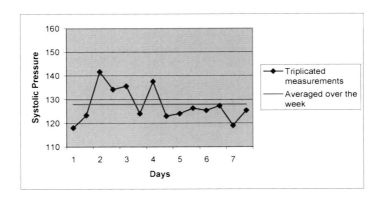

Figure 24. Calculation of average systolic blood pressure from forty-two of fifty-six measurements collected over seven days.

OPTION FOUR

Upward drift of usual blood pressure can be detected by weekly measurements at the end of each month (See Figure 25). Although no trend is revealed by measurements between months 6 to 9, a progressive rise is apparent from measurements taken over a longer period.

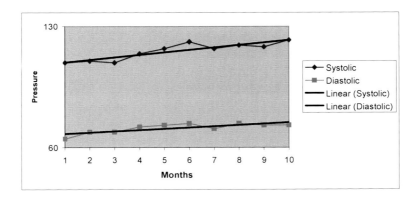

Figure 25. Detection of an upward trend by measurement of averaged systolic pressure each month

OPTION FIVE

Successive weekly measurements can be used to detect changes that result from treatment. For instance, there is a gradual decline of usual blood pressure following introduction of a diuretic (See Figure 26). Following the occurrence of symptomatic gout, the diuretic was withdrawn. This resulted in a prompt rise of pressure over a period of four weeks, which clearly exceeds levels recommended by the Mayo Clinic (See Figure 27). Reintroduction of the usual dose of diuretic halted this rise, although eight weeks had to elapse before control of blood pressure was fully restored. Use of a reduced dose of diuretic was attempted, but was abandoned because loss of control was also unacceptable (See Figure 28).

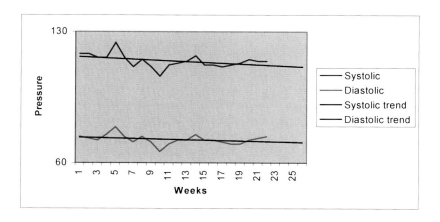

Figure 26. Weekly measurement of blood pressure following introduction of a diuretic. The trend lines reveal a progressive reduction of pressure.

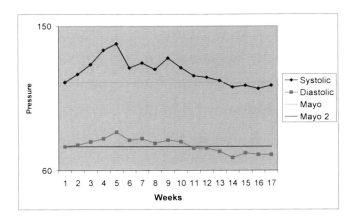

Figure 27. Withdrawal of a diuretic between weeks 0 and 4 results in a loss of blood pressure control that persists for some time after reintroduction of the diuretic.

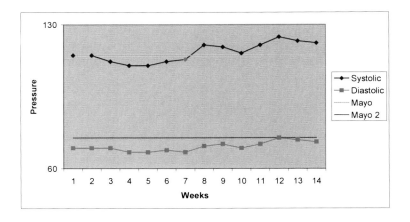

Figure 28. Weekly measurement of blood pressure when using a diuretic at a normal dose (weeks 1-7) and at half of this dose (week 8 onwards)

8. Who can benefit from self-measurement?

Individuals for whom diagnosis of high blood pressure has been considered
Patients who are being treated for high blood pressure
Patients who have already had a stroke or a coronary heart attack
Patients with diabetes
Pregnant women
Individuals whose usual blood pressure exceeds 115 (systolic) or 75 (diastolic) mm of mercury

ressures that consistently exceed 140 (systolic) or 90 (diastolic) mm of mercury
~e diagnostic for high blood pressure. Because of day to day variation, high
lood pressure can easily be overlooked when making measurements in isolation.
uch oversight may be avoided by calculating averaged blood pressure from
plicate measurements. As replication is time consuming, the limitations of
litary measurements are often disregarded during clinical consultation. For
istance, guidelines on "Management of hypertension in adults in primary care"
om the National Institute for Clinical Excellence recommend that a general
ractitioner should make a single measurement at the onset of a consultation if
atients are not known to have high blood pressure. Expansion to a second
ieasurement at the end of the consultation would depend upon whether the first
ieasurement indicted high blood pressure and whether there was sufficient time.
iould high blood pressure be detected by the first measurement and then
onfirmed by a second measurement, additional paired measurements would
ave to be made on three separate occasions. If following this protocol, diagnosis
ecomes critically dependent upon the initial measurement and it would not be
xceptional for such isolated measurements to be misleading. In this way, high
ood pressure might remain undetected for some time since guidelines
commend a further measurement at sometime within the next five years. It is
ierefore fortunate that the relatively complex procedure of blood pressure
ieasurement in the clinic has effectively become automated. By using an
itomated procedure for self-measurement, it is possible to escape from time
onstraints that govern many activities within a clinic. This makes detection of
gh blood pressure inescapable and allows control to be monitored easily during

treatment. Possibly of greater importance, regular self-measurement allows any trend towards high blood pressure to be detected at an early stage.

Patients whose high blood pressure has been diagnosed should not allow their usual blood pressure to exceed 138.5 (systolic) and 82.6 (diastolic) mm of mercury. For, once these thresholds are breached, the risk of strokes and coronary heart attacks will rise progressively. Before diagnosis of increased blood pressure the corresponding thresholds are pressures of 115 (systolic) and 75 (diastolic) mm of mercury. As for high blood pressure, the increased risk of strokes and coronary heart attacks reflects usual blood pressure as pressures rise above these thresholds. Once pressure has risen into the pre-hypertensive range of 115-14 (systolic) and 75-90 (diastolic) mm of mercury, it is debatable whether these increased risks are lost if usual pressures revert to less than 115 (systolic) and 7 (diastolic) mm of mercury. As both raised blood pressure and increased risk c strokes or coronary heart attacks are eliminated by termination of pregnancy, it i possible that changes could offer protection. This inference is reinforced by a increased survival of diabetic patients on lowering blood pressure. Nonetheless, i cannot be presumed that increased vulnerability to strokes and coronary heart attacks is wholly excluded by restoring usual blood pressure to 115 (systolic) an 75 (diastolic) mm of mercury. On balance, reducing blood pressure by a change c lifestyle or use of drugs to lower blood pressure will prevent increased risk ye may be modestly effective in reversing those changes that underlie increase vulnerability during pre-hypertension.

As blood pressure rises, the likelihood of a blockage of arterial vessels increase thereby making strokes or coronary heart attacks more frequent during hig blood pressure. It has long been recognised that individuals who have alread experienced such misfortune are susceptible to a further episode. Survey of suc patients reveals a mortality of 5% each year, which is ten-fold greater than fc comparable individuals who have not previously experienced a stroke or coronary heart attack. Detection of poor control in such patients is therefor particularly important and self-measurement provides a simple method fc regular monitoring. If blood pressures remain controlled and usual bloo pressure is not rising, self-measurement will be reassuring. If pressures closel approach or exceed thresholds used for diagnosis of high blood pressure or pressures exceed target levels set by an adviser, clinical reassessment will be needed.

Arterial vessels in diabetic individuals may be more susceptible to rupture or blockage because of exaggerated stiffness of the vessel wall in areas affected by arteriosclerosis. Increased susceptibility to strokes and coronary heart disease is therefore a major hazard for patients with diabetes, whose vulnerability increases as blood pressure rises. For this reason, it is usual for diabetic patients to attempt to maintain their blood pressure at less than 130 (systolic) and at less than 80 (diastolic) mm of mercury. Even at these lower pressures, diabetic patients have a risk of strokes and coronary heart attacks that is greater than the risk in comparable individuals who are not diabetic. To confer maximal protection, it is therefore desirable to lower resting blood pressure even further. Adhering to such advice necessitates very close monitoring of usual blood pressure and regular self-measurement would seem to be the only way of achieving this objective.

High blood pressure is a feature of one in every ten pregnancies. For this reason, blood pressure is monitored routinely as part of antenatal care. Regular measurement of blood pressure by the midwife detects this complication of pregnancy efficiently and allows complications to be avoided. However, there may be circumstances (e.g. travelling, staff changes, transport difficulties) that interrupt regular monitoring. Self-measurement provides a simple way to circumvent such discontinuity and to avoid loss of data. The objective of routine measurement of blood pressure in pregnancy is to detect any upward trend. Such a trend will become apparent earlier, and onset will be detected with greater certainty, if self-measurements are made frequently. Hence, daily self-measurement can provide a more sensitive indication of the onset of an upward trend than infrequent measurements during antenatal examinations. In pregnancy, early detection of an upward trend by self-measurement is therefore an advantage. Set against this advantage is the finding that some oscillometric measurements can be less precise in pregnancy. Even so, self-measurement should enable a mother to detect an upward trend and alert her to seek more comprehensive clinical examination.

In developed countries, blood pressures in the region of 100 (systolic) and 60 (diastolic) mm of mercury are not exceptional in persons who are young and healthy. However, such individuals will almost invariably experience a remorseless rise of blood pressure with age. Once over 60, less than 1% will have a systolic blood pressure of 100 mm of mercury, whereas more than 70% will have a systolic blood pressure that already exceeds 140 mm of mercury. These elevated systolic pressures predict an increased risk of strokes and coronary heart attacks. Such misfortune is not confined to those whose systolic pressures exceed 140 mm of mercury since the risk of strokes and coronary heart attacks is increased for all levels of systolic pressure in excess of 115 mm of mercury. Until relatively recently, pressures of 120 (systolic) and 80 (diastolic) mm of mercury were considered optimal and without increased hazard. However, it is now recognised that even these pressures are associated with significantly increased risks of strokes and coronary heart attack. Hence, if self-measurement detects pressures above 115 (systolic) or 75 (diastolic) mm of mercury, it is worthwhile to give serious consideration to lifestyle changes that might avoid, or at least retard, progression towards high blood pressure. Self-measurement provides a simple and convenient monitoring system whereby those who favour preventive maintenance can appraise their current status and can anticipate deterioration by monitoring progression of their blood pressure over long periods.

Most adults will know how much they weigh and many will monitor their body weight in the bathroom on a daily or weekly basis. Even though high blood pressure is a frequent consequence of excessive body weight, few will be aware of their usual blood pressure, let alone be making regular measurements. If such individuals were to measure blood pressure routinely, they might benefit by detecting the onset of permanently raised blood pressure. Pressures in excess of 115 (systolic) or 75 (diastolic) mm of mercury are now recognised as precursors of high blood pressure. In the USA, this finding has led to suggestion that blood pressures should be measured every two years from age 21 onwards. The "Seventh Report of the Joint National Committee on Prevention, Detection, Evaluation and Treatment of High Blood Pressure" emphasises a need for prevention. Current evidence indicates that pressures of 120 (systolic) and 80 (diastolic) mm of mercury are not low enough to avoid serious consequences of high blood pressure. The committee therefore recommends that individuals whose systolic blood pressure has reached 115 mm of mercury should monitor their usual blood pressure at regular intervals. Because of the very large numbers at risk, self-measurement is the only realistic way of adhering to such advice.

9. Selected sources of information

As you may wish to explore aspects of high blood pressure that are covered in the text, some source references are listed. Abstracts of these publications and, in some instances, copies of the complete publication can be obtained without charge by using the Internet.

Measurement of blood pressure

Recommendations for blood pressure measurement in humans and experimental animals.
Pickering and others: Hypertension (2005) volume 45, pages 142-161.
[A survey of the advantages and limitations of methods for measurement of blood pressure that are in current use]

Measurement of blood pressure: an evidence-based review.
McAlister and Straus: British Medical Journal (2001) volume 322, pages 908-911.
[Discussion of factors that influence the precision of measurement]

User procedure for self-measurement of blood pressure. First International Consensus Conference on Self Blood Pressure Measurement.
Mengden and others: Blood Pressure Monitoring (2000) volume 5, pages 111-129.
[Technical recommendations for self-measurement]

Risk of strokes and coronary heart attacks

Impact of high-normal blood pressure on the risk of cardiovascular disease.
Vasan and others: New England Journal of Medicine (2001) volume 345, pages 1291-1297.
[Analysis of the fate of 6859 participants from the Framingham Heart Study. These subjects were not diagnosed with high blood pressure yet experienced increased cardiovascular disease]

Age-specific relevance of usual blood pressure to vascular mortality: a meta-analysis of individual data for one million adults in 61 prospective studies.
Lewington and others: Lancet (2002) volume 360, pages 1903-1913.
[Throughout middle and old age, mortality is directly proportional to usual blood pressure for systolic pressures above 115 mm of mercury and for diastolic pressures above 75 mm of mercury]

Essential hypertension.
Messerli and others: Lancet (2007) volume 370, pages 591-603.
[Review giving perspective to the measurement, cardiovascular consequences and treatment of high blood pressure]

Mechanisms of thrombogenesis in atrial fibrillation: Virchow's triad revisited.
Watson and others: Lancet (2009) volume 373, pages 155-166.
[An overview of mechanisms that underlie arterial blockade, giving emphasis to the role of arterial thrombi as a precursor of strokes]

Treatment with drugs that lower blood pressure

Initial treatment of hypertension.
August: New England Journal of Medicine (2003) volume 348, pages 610-617.
[Description of the strategy followed in treating a new case of high blood pressure in USA]

Usual versus tight control of systolic blood pressure in non-diabetic patients with hypertension (Cardio-Sis): an open-label randomised trial.
Verdecchia and others: Lancet (2009) volume 374, pages 525-533.
[Reveals protection from ventricular hypertrophy by setting 130 mm of mercury as a target for systolic pressure contol]

Effects of a polypill (Polycap) on risk factors in middle-aged individuals without cardiovascular disease (TIPS): a phase II, double-blind, randomised trial.
The Indian Polycap Study (TIPS): Lancet (2009) volume 373, pages 1341-1351.
[Combining three blood pressure lowering drugs with a statin, aspirin and folic acid reduces the likelihood of cardiovascular events (blood pressure, heart rate, blood lipids and platelet activation)]

Antihypertensive drugs.
Kaplan and Opie: In "Drugs for the Heart" 7th edition (2009) Eds L.H.Opie &
B.J.Gersh. Saunders/Elsevier
An expert overview of the pharmacology of hypertension]

Modifying lifestyle to lower blood pressure

National Heart, Lung and Blood Institute Workshop on sodium and blood
pressure: a critical review of current scientific evidence.
Chobanian and Hill: Hypertension (2000) volume 35, pages 858-863.
Consensus of expert opinion]

Weight threshold and blood pressure in a lean black population.
Junker and others: Hypertension (1995) volume 26, pages 616-623.
Blood pressure level rises when BMI exceeds a threshold of 21.5 kg/m^2]

Obesity-associated hypertension and kidney disease.
Current Opinions in Nephrology and Hypertension (2003) volume 12, pages 195-
00.
Excess weight gain may be responsible for 65-75% of the risk for high blood
pressure. Describes a mechanism to account for this interrelationship]

ffect of dietary patterns on ambulatory blood pressure: results from the dietary
approaches to stop hypertension (DASH) trial.
Moore and others: Hypertension (1999) volume 34, pages 472-477.
Demonstrates that the DASH combination diet reduces blood pressure,
specially in patients with high blood pressure]

Results of the Diet, Exercise and Weight Loss Intervention Trial (DEW-IT).
Miller and others: Hypertension (2002) volume 40, pages 612-618.
Inclusion of exercise with the DASH diet lowers blood pressure]

Blood pressure in non-acculturated societies

Blood pressure, sodium intake and sodium related hormones in the Yanomamo Indians, a "no-salt" culture.
Oliver and others: Circulation (1975) volume 52, pages 146-151.
[The presence of increased amounts of renin and aldosterone in blood during avoidance of salt implies that their secretion is being suppressed by dietary salt in urban populations]

Cardiovascular risk factors in a Melanesian population apparently free from stroke and ischaemic heart disease: the Kitava study.
Lindberg and others: Journal of Internal Medicine (1994) volume 236, pages 331-340.
[Comparison with Europeans implies that leanness and low blood pressure explains the absence of stroke and coronary heart attacks]

The rocky road from roots to rice: a review of the changing food and nutrition situation in Papua New Guinea.
Saweri: Papua New Guinea Medical Journal (2001) volume 44, pages 151-163.
[Increased incidence of high blood pressure and coronary heart disease when villagers adopt an urban lifestyle in which there is a high-energy diet]

High blood pressure in diabetes

Diabetes running wild
Diamond: Nature (1992) volume 357, pages 362-363.
[Diabetes epidemic when Narau islanders became wealthy and adopted a sedentary lifestyle, eating high-energy foods in place of fishing and farming.]

Improving microvascular outcomes in patients with diabetes through management of hypertension.
McGill: Postgraduate Medicine (2009) volume 121, pages 89-101.
[Treatment of high blood pressure and hyperglycaemia to limit retinopathy and nephropathy]

Usefulness of home blood pressure measurement in the morning in type 2 diabetic patients.
Kamoi and others: Diabetes Care (2002) volume 25, pages 2218-2223.

[Recommendation of self-measurement in the morning to minimise vessel damage and consequent increased mortality]

High blood pressure in arteriosclerosis

From vulnerable plaque to vulnerable patient.
Naghavi and others: Circulation (2003) volume 108, pages 1772-1778.
[Explains current strategies for detecting plaque and amongst patients who are vulnerable to occlusion of coronary vessels]

Endothelial therapy of atherosclerosis and its risk factors.
Traupe and others: Current Research in Vascular Pharmacology (2003) volume 1, pages 111-121.
[How therapy for high blood pressure might improve endothelial function]

High blood pressure and insulin

Low serum insulin in traditional Pacific Islanders - the Kitava study.
Lindberg and others: Metabolism (1999) volume 48, pages 116-1219.
[In Pacific Islanders, the amount of insulin in serum is low and declines with age. In a comparable Swedish population amounts are higher and rise with age]

Prevalence of the metabolic syndrome among US adults: findings from the third National Heath and Nutrition Examination Survey.
Ford and others: Journal of the American Medical Association (2002) volume 287, pages 356-359.
[High blood pressure is a feature of the 47 million residents in USA who were affected by the metabolic syndrome in 2000]

High blood pressure in pregnancy

High sensitivity test for the early diagnosis of gestational hypertension and pre-eclampsia.

Hermida and others: Journal of Perinatal Medicine (1997) volume 25, pages 101-109.
[In normal delivery, there is a fall of blood pressure until week 20 followed by a rise until delivery. In gestational hypertension and pre-eclampsia there is a continuous linear increase until termination]

Automated self-initiated blood pressure or 24-hour ambulatory blood pressure monitoring in pregnancy?
Brown and others: British Journal of Obstetrics and Gynaecology (2004) volume 111, pages 38-41.
[Use of Omron 705CP to eliminate "white coat effect" in pregnant women]

An accurate automated blood pressure device for use in pregnancy and pre-eclampsia: the Microlife 3BTO-A.
Reinders and others: British Journal of Obstetrics and Gynaecology (2005) volume 112, pages 915-920.
[Evaluation of the accuracy of the Microlife 3BTO-A, a self-measurement device in normal pregnancy as well as pregnancy accompanied by high blood pressure or by pre-eclampsia]